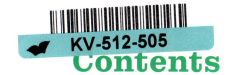

Contents

Chapter 1: What is Cancer?

Chapter 2: Signs & Symptoms

Chapter 3: Diagnosis & Treatment

Introduction

Cancer is Volume 433 in the **issues** series. The aim of the series is to offer current, diverse information about important issues in our world, from a UK perspective.

About Cancer

1 in 2 people will develop some form of cancer during their lifetime. Almost all of us know someone who has been affected by cancer. This book looks at causes and types of cancer, diagnosis, treatments and how to self-examine.

Our sources

Titles in the **issues** series are designed to function as educational resource books, providing a balanced overview of a specific subject.

The information in our books is comprised of facts, articles and opinions from many different sources, including:

- Newspaper reports and opinion pieces
- Website factsheets
- Magazine and journal articles
- Statistics and surveys
- Government reports
- Literature from special interest groups.

A note on critical evaluation

Because the information reprinted here is from a number of different sources, readers should bear in mind the origin of the text and whether the source is likely to have a particular bias when presenting information (or when conducting their research). It is hoped that, as you read about the many aspects of the issues explored in this book, you will critically evaluate the information presented.

It is important that you decide whether you are being presented with facts or opinions. Does the writer give a biased or unbiased report? If an opinion is being expressed, do you agree with the writer? Is there potential bias to the 'facts' or statistics behind an article?

Activities

Throughout this book, you will find a selection of assignments and activities designed to help you engage with the articles you have been reading and to explore your own opinions. Some tasks will take longer than others and there is a mixture of design, writing and research-based activities that you can complete alone or in a group.

Further research

At the end of each article we have listed its source and a website that you can visit if you would like to conduct your own research. Please remember to critically evaluate any sources that you consult and consider whether the information you are viewing is accurate and unbiased.

Issues Online

The **issues** series of books is complemented by our online resource, issuesonline.co.uk

On the Issues Online website you will find a wealth of information, covering over 70 topics, to support the PSHE and RSE curriculum.

Why Issues Online?

Researching a topic? Issues Online is the best place to start for...

Librarians

Issues Online is an essential tool for librarians: feel confident you are signposting safe, reliable, user-friendly online resources to students and teaching staff alike. We provide multi-user concurrent access, so no waiting around for another student to finish with a resource. Issues Online also provides FREE downloadable posters for your shelf/wall/table displays.

Teachers

Issues Online is an ideal resource for lesson planning, inspiring lively debate in class and setting lessons and homework tasks.

Our accessible, engaging content helps deepen students' knowledge, promotes critical thinking and develops independent learning skills.

Issues Online saves precious preparation time. We wade through the wealth of material on the internet to filter the best quality, most relevant and up-to-date information you need to start exploring a topic.

Our carefully selected, balanced content presents an overview and insight into each topic from a variety of sources and viewpoints.

Students

Issues Online is designed to support your studies in a broad range of topics, particularly social issues relevant to young people today.

Thousands of articles, statistics and infographs instantly available to help you with research and assignments.

With 24/7 access using the powerful Algolia search system, you can find relevant information quickly, easily and safely anytime from your laptop, tablet or smartphone, in class or at home.

Visit issuesonline.co.uk to find out more!

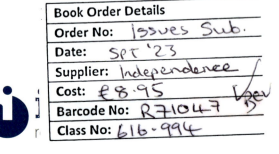

Book Order Details	
Order No:	Issues Sub.
Date:	Sep '23
Supplier:	Independence
Cost:	£8.95
Barcode No:	R71047
Class No:	616.994

raries

What is Cancer?

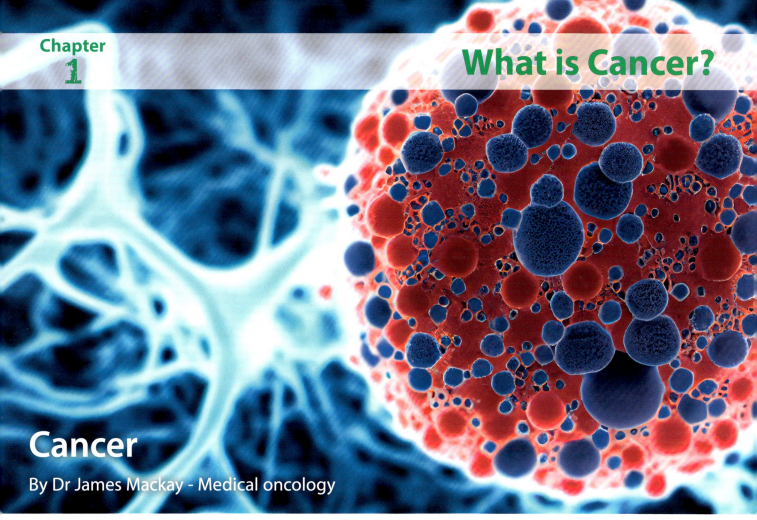

Cancer

By Dr James Mackay - Medical oncology

What is cancer?

Cancer occurs when cells, which are the building blocks of the tissues and organs in the body, begin to grow uncontrollably. The body's control mechanism stops working and the old cells do not die but instead, grow out of control. They then form a mass of tissue known as a tumour, which can be benign (non-cancerous) or malignant (cancerous). There are some cancers, such as leukaemia, which do not manifest as a tumour.

Cancer can form anywhere on the body. Some types of cancer grow and quickly invade other parts of the body to form new tumours (a process called metastasis), while others remain confined to their place of origin. Benign cancers, for example, won't usually develop metastasis.

It is estimated that one in three men and one in four women will be affected by cancer over the course of their lifetime.

What are the different groups of cancer?

Cancer which form in specific types of cells can be divided into five categories:

1. Carcinomas:

Forming in the epithelial cells (cells that surround the body's surface), carcinomas are the most common type of cancer. The four different types of carcinomas are: adenocarcinoma (most of breast, colon and prostate cancers); basal cell carcinoma (skin cancer); squamous cell carcinoma (other type of skin cancer); and transitional cell carcinoma (some bladder, ureters and kidney cancers).

2. Lymphomas:

Developing in the lymphocytes (a white blood cell), lymphomas usually build up in the lymph nodes in the neck. The two main types of lymphomas are Hodgkin lymphomas (formed from B-cells) and non-Hodgkin lymphomas (formed from B-cells or T-cells).

3. Leukaemias:

Beginning in the bone marrow, leukaemias don't form tumours. Instead, large quantities of abnormal white blood cells build up in the bloodstream and bone marrow, forcing out healthy blood cells. The four types of leukaemias are: chronic lymphocytic leukaemia, acute myeloid leukaemia, chronic myeloid leukaemia and acute lymphocytic leukaemia.

Leukaemias are classified as either acute (fast-growing) or chronic (slow-growing). They are also named by the type of white blood cells affected: lymphocytic (developed in the lymphocytes) or myeloid (developed in red blood cells, platelets and other white blood cells - excepting lymphocytes).

4. Brain tumours:

They can form in any part of the brain, including the skull base, the brainstem, the sinuses and the nasal cavity. However, it is important to know that not all brain tumours are cancerous.

Benign brain tumours grow very slowly, with distinct borders and rarely spread. They are still dangerous, however. The most common types of benign brain tumours are: meningiomas, pituitary adenomas and schwannomas.

On the other hand, malignant brain tumours are cancerous, grow quickly and invade nearby brain structures. The most common types of malignant brain tumours include gliomas, medulloblastoma and astrocytomas.

5. Sarcomas:

Originating in the bone and soft tissue (including muscles, connective tissue, blood vessels and ligaments), sarcomas are the rarest type of cancer. There are more than 70 different types of sarcomas, all of which differ depending on the location of their place of origin. Osteosarcoma, for example, forms in the bones; liposarcoma in the fat and rhabdomyosarcoma in the muscles.

What are the symptoms?

Cancer can cause various symptoms, but in many cases, these symptoms won't be related to cancer at all and instead be caused by other conditions. They may also vary depending on the type and location of the tumour.

Common signs and symptoms associated with cancer include:

- Persistent fevers or sweats
- Changes in the skin, such as yellowing, darkening or redness
- Changes in weight
- Unexplained bleeding
- Changes in your bowel habits
- A sudden lump or thickening under the skin
- Persistent cough or breathing problems
- Difficulty swallowing

Seek medical attention if you experience persistent changes in your body's natural processes or unusual, sudden symptoms. These can be an early sign of cancer.

What is cancer staging?

Staging is used to describe the size of cancer and how far it has grown. It is also important as it enables your doctor and cancer care team to understand what type of treatment plan you will need to follow. Different types of exams which include CT scans, MRIs, endoscopies, biopsies and lab tests, will help to determine the stage of your cancer.

There are two parts to cancer staging: the TNM system and the number.

TNM stands for 'tumour, nodule, metastasis.' It recognises the size of the initial cancer tumour (called the primary tumour), whether it has spread to the nearby lymph nodes and if it has spread to other parts of the body. During the TNM, your doctor will also check for other tumours nearby.

The numbers are used to divide cancer into its stage, as follows:

- Stage 1: the cancer is small and contained within the area that it started.
- Stage 2: the tumour is larger but has not yet started to spread into nearby tissues. Sometimes it might have spread into the lymph nodes.
- Stage 3: the cancer is larger and may have spread into the surrounding tissues and into the lymph nodes.
- Stage 4: it has spread into a distant organ in the body. It can also be called advanced or metastatic cancer.

In most cases, cancer is staged during its diagnosis, although in some cases it can be staged again (called restaging) after the start of treatment or if the cancer recurs.

With restaging, the new information will be added on to the original stage without replacing it. Even if it worsens or spreads, a cancer will always be referred to the stage it was appointed at diagnosis. This is done to help your doctor understand your medical progress, the prognosis and learn how different patients respond to treatment.

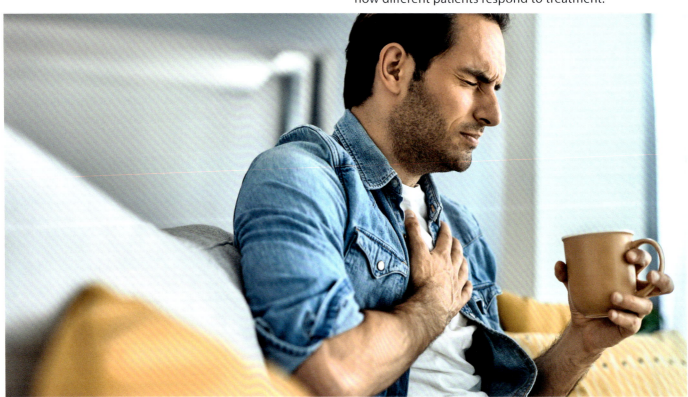

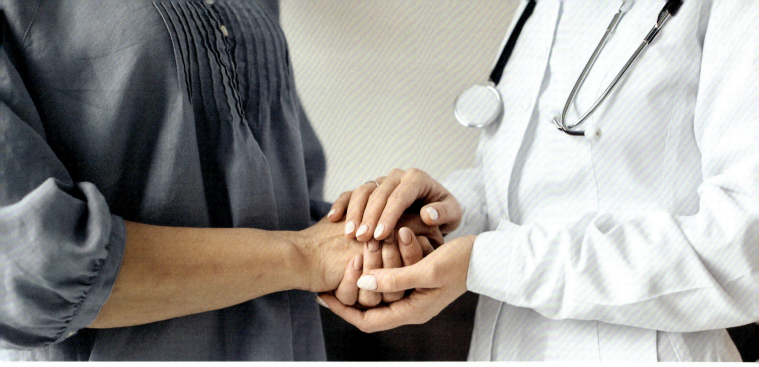

What are the most common types of cancer?

In the UK, the most common types of cancer are:

- Breast cancer
- Lung cancer
- Prostate cancer
- Bowel cancer

There are more than 200 types of cancer and each one is diagnosed and treated in a different way.

How is cancer treated?

The treatment of cancer depends on your individual case, including the stage that you have been diagnosed with. Some types of cancer will require a combination of treatments.

Surgery is usually the first part of the treatment plan in order to resect (remove) solid tumours if these haven't spread to other parts of the body and remain in one area. Skin cancers, lung cancers and breast cancers are usually treated this way.

If the tumour has spread to the nearby lymph nodes, these may be extracted to remove the tumour from the body.

In some cases, complete removal of the tumour may not be possible, for example if it has spread to sensitive areas of the body. In this case, the surgeon will remove as much of the tumour as possible and your doctor will then recommend chemotherapy and/or radiotherapy.

Chemotherapy, which uses drugs to kill cancer cells, can be given intravenously into the vein or orally with tablets. Eat well and take time to rest if you're undergoing chemotherapy treatment. Avoid people who are sick with a cold or the flu, as chemotherapy will debilitate your immune system.

In radiotherapy, radiation is used to kill the cancer cells and can be given in a number of ways, such as via a machine beaming radiation at the cancer site, or via radiotherapy injections into the blood.

Other types of cancer treatment include: bone marrow transplant which uses higher doses of chemotherapy; immunotherapy which helps your body's immune system fight the cancer; hormone therapy which removes or blocks cancer-fuelling hormones from the body, and targeted drug therapy.

Are cancerous lumps hard or painful?

Cancerous lumps are generally large, hard, sudden and painless to the touch. Those that can be felt from the outside of the body can appear in your neck, breasts, testicles, arms and legs. As weeks pass, the lump(s) may steadily increase in size.

Is cancer genetic?

Cancer is a disease caused by changes (mutations) to the DNA within the cells of our body. These mutations, which affect a cell's normal functions of growth and division, can instruct a healthy cell to stop preventing uncontrolled cell growth and stop repairing DNA errrors. These can cause a cell to become cancerous.

In regards to family history, you may be born with gene mutations that you inherited from your parents. However, this type of mutation only accounts for a small percentage of cancers. The majority of gene mutations that cause cancer are acquired after birth through smoking, radiation, viruses, chronic inflammation and a lack of exercise.

What happens if cancer recurs?

Cancer may come back if some cancer cells remain in your body, despite treatment. A cancer recurrence can occur in the same place where your cancer first developed or in another part of the body.

In these cases, treatment will be different from the first time as tumours that recur don't respond to treatment the same way as the initial tumour did, due to cancer cells becoming more resistant to chemotherapy.

2 December 2019

www.topdoctors.co.uk

How cancer starts

Cell changes and cancer

All cancers begin in cells. Our bodies are made up of more than a hundred million million (100,000,000,000,000) cells. Cancer starts with changes in one cell or a small group of cells.

Usually, we have just the right number of each type of cell. This is because cells produce signals to control how much and how often the cells divide. If any of these signals are faulty or missing, cells might start to grow and multiply too much and form a lump called a tumour.

A primary tumour is where the cancer starts. Some types of cancer, called leukaemia , start from blood cells. They don't form solid tumours. Instead, the cancer cells build up in the blood and sometimes the bone marrow

For a cancer to start, certain changes take place within the genes of a cell or a group of cells.

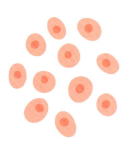

Normal cells

- Uniform cell shape
- Spheroid shape, single nucleus
- Large cytoplasmic volume
- Controlled growth
- Remain in their intended location

Cancer cells

- Irregular cell shape and size
- Multiple irregular shape nucleus
- Small cytoplasmic volume
- Uncontrolled growth
- Can spread to different locations (metastasis)

Genes and cell division

Different types of cells in the body do different jobs. But they are basically similar.

All cells have a control centre called a nucleus. Inside the nucleus are chromosomes made up of thousands of genes. Genes contain long strings of DNA (deoxyribonucleic acid), which are coded messages that tell the cell how to behave.

Each gene is an instruction that tells the cell to make something. This could be a protein or a different type of molecule called RNA (ribonucleic acid). Together, proteins and RNA control the cell. They decide:

- what sort of cell it will be
- what it does
- when it divides
- when it dies

Gene changes within cells (mutations)

Genes make sure that cells grow and make copies (reproduce) in an orderly and controlled way. And are needed to keep the body healthy.

Sometimes a change happens in the genes when a cell divides. This is a mutation. It means that a gene has been damaged or lost or copied too many times.

Mutations can happen by chance when a cell is dividing. Some mutations mean that the cell no longer understands its instructions. It can start to grow out of control. There have to be about 6 different mutations before a normal cell turns into a cancer cell.

Mutations in particular genes may mean that:

- a cell starts making too many proteins that trigger a cell to divide
- a cell stops making proteins that normally tell a cell to stop dividing
- abnormal proteins may be produced that work differently to normal

It can take many years for a damaged cell to divide and grow and form a tumour big enough to cause symptoms or show up on a scan.

How mutations happen

Mutations can happen by chance when a cell is dividing. They can also be caused by the processes of life inside the cell. Or by things coming from outside the body, such as the chemicals in tobacco smoke. And some people can inherit faults in particular genes that make them more likely to develop a cancer.

Some genes get damaged every day and cells are very good at repairing them. But over time, the damage may build up. And once cells start growing too fast, they are more likely to pick up further mutations and less likely to be able to repair the damaged genes.

1 July 2020

www.cancerresearchuk.org

Causes and risk factors

There are things that can increase your risk of getting cancer. Find out what these might be and the possible changes you could make to reduce your risk.

What are risk factors?

Everyone has a certain risk of developing cancer. A combination of genes, lifestyle and environment can affect this risk. Doctors do not know the exact causes of cancer. But there are risk factors that can increase your chance of developing it.

Having one or more risk factors does not mean you will get cancer. Also, having no risk factors does not mean you will not develop cancer.

Around 1 in 3 cases of the most common cancers (about 33%) could be prevented by eating a healthy diet, keeping to a healthy weight and being more active. There are some things you can do to lower your risk of developing cancer. But you cannot reduce your risk completely through your lifestyle.

Age

For most people, increasing age is the biggest risk factor for developing cancer. In general, people over 65 have the greatest risk of developing cancer. People under 50 have a much lower risk.

Family history

Cancer is very common and most of us have relatives who have had cancer. People often worry that a history of cancer in their family greatly increases their risk of developing it. But fewer than 1 in 10 cancers are associated with a strong family history of cancer. If you are worried, you should talk to your GP.

Lifestyle risk factors and reducing your risk

Giving up smoking

In the UK, more than 1 in 4 cancer deaths (over 25%) are caused by smoking.

Breathing in other people's smoke (passive smoking) also increases your risk of developing cancer.

Keep your home smoke-free to protect you and your family's health. If you smoke, giving up is one of the most important thing you can do for your health.

If you want to give up smoking, it is never too late to stop. Ask your GP for advice, or contact the stop-smoking service in your area.

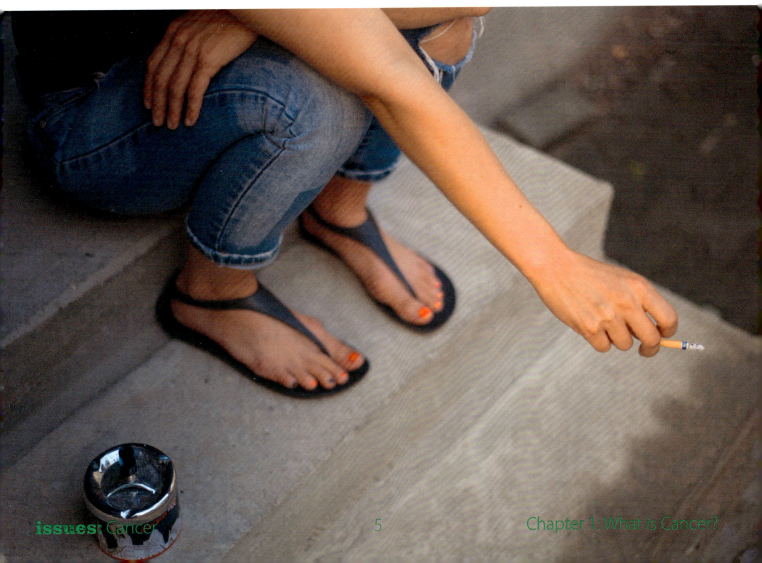

Keeping to a healthy weight

Being overweight increases the risk of many types of cancer, including cancers of the bowel, kidney, womb and gullet (oesophagus). Women who are overweight and have been through the menopause also have a higher risk of breast cancer.

Keeping to a healthy body weight reduces your risk of cancer and other health problems, such as heart disease and diabetes.

If you are worried about your weight or need more information, talk to your GP or a dietitian.

Eating a balanced diet

There is no single food that causes or prevents cancer.

Eating a balanced diet is good for your overall health and helps reduce your risk of some cancers. It can also help you to keep to a healthy weight.

Eating plenty of high-fibre foods helps reduce the risk of bowel cancer. Red and processed meat are linked to a higher risk of bowel and prostate cancer. Try to limit how much you eat. Red meats include beef, pork, lamb and veal. Processed meats include sausages, bacon, salami, tinned meats, and packet meats like sandwich ham.

Being physically active

Many studies have found that regular physical activity can reduce the risk of cancer. You should try to do at least 30 minutes of activity every day.

Your cancer risk is reduced further if you are active for more than 30 minutes a day and if you exercise harder (vigorous activity). The NHS has more information on how to stay active.

Limiting how much alcohol you drink

Drinking alcohol increases your risk of mouth and throat cancers. But it is also linked to other cancers.

In general, the more you drink, the higher your risk. Your risk is even higher if you also smoke.

You should try to stick to the current guidelines on drinking alcohol.

Taking care in the sun

Spending some time outside in the sun helps you stay healthy. Our bodies need sunlight to make vitamin D.

But it is important to protect your skin from burning, as this can increase your risk of skin cancers.

If you are going to be out in the sun for longer than a few minutes, you should protect your skin:

- Keep your arms and legs covered by wearing long-sleeved tops and trousers. Wear a wide-brimmed hat to protect your face and neck.

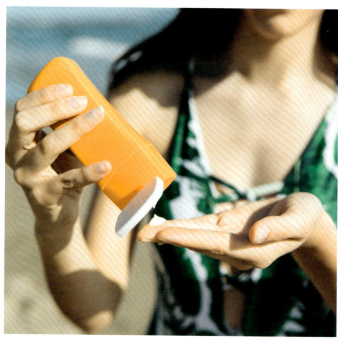

- Use suncream with a high sun protection factor (SPF) of at least 30. Choose one that protects against UVA and UVB, with four or five stars.

- Make sure you use enough sun cream. Experts say you need at least six to eight teaspoons of lotion for an average-sized adult to give the SPF coverage it says on the bottle.

- Stay out of the sun during the hottest part of the day. This is usually between 11am and 3pm.

Using sun beds or sun lamps also increases your risk of skin cancer. If you want to look tanned, use fake-tanning lotions or sprays.

Other risk factors

Workplace and environmental factors

Exposure to harmful substances in the environment or workplace can cause cancer. Substances that cause cancer are called carcinogens. Some of these carcinogens can cause cancer years after you have been exposed to them.

If you have a cancer caused by your workplace, you may be able to claim Industrial Injuries Disablement Benefit.

Asbestos

Asbestos is a natural mineral that is now banned in the UK. It can damage the lungs and cause mesothelioma. The people most likely to have been exposed to asbestos at work include people who work in construction, ship and boiler makers. People who have not worked with asbestos may also be at risk. This can happen if they have been exposed to asbestos factories, buildings that contain asbestos or if they live with someone working with asbestos.

Chemicals

Some chemicals have been linked to bladder cancer. The chemicals were previously used in dye factories and other industries. Many of these chemicals are now banned. But bladder cancer can take more than 25 years to develop after you are exposed to the chemicals. Some chemicals can also slightly increase the risk of skin cancer. Many of these chemicals are also banned.

Environmental causes

One of the main environmental causes of cancer is ultraviolet (UV) radiation from the sun. We know that many skin cancers, including melanoma, are caused by spending too much time in the sun. The people most at risk are those who work outside, and those who are fair-skinned. There are things you can do to reduce your risk (see above).

Radon is another possible source of radiation that may be linked to cancer. Radon is a natural gas that is found in rock in parts of the UK. Radon has been linked to lung cancer. But the risk is very small.

Low immunity

If you have low immunity, your immune system does not work as well. This means you are more likely to get infections.

People with a lower immunity may have:

- had a transplant and take drugs to suppress the immune system – these drugs stop the body rejecting the transplant
- HIV (human immunodeficiency virus)
- a medical condition that lowers their immunity.

If you have low immunity, you may be more likely to develop some cancers. These cancers include lymphoma, non-melanoma skin cancer and Kaposi's sarcoma, or cancers caused by a virus or bacteria.

Viruses and bacteria

Viral infections are very common and usually do not cause cancer to develop. A small number of viruses have been linked to a higher risk of certain types of cancer. These include:

Human papilloma viruses (HPV)

HPV increases the risk of cervical cancer and has also been linked to some other cancers.

Epstein-Barr virus

This is linked to some types of lymphoma.

Hepatitis B and C

These viruses have been linked to liver cancer.

HIV

This can increase the risk of cancers including lymphoma and sarcoma.

T-cell leukaemia virus

This is linked to T-cell leukaemia in adults.

Key Facts

- Around 1 in 3 cases of the most common cancers (about 33%) could be prevented by eating a healthy diet, keeping to a healthy weight and being more active.

- Fewer than 1 in 10 cancers are associated with a strong family history of cancer.

- People over 65 have the greatest risk of developing cancer. People under 50 have a much lower risk.

- More than 1 in 4 cancer deaths (over 25%) are caused by smoking.

There is also a common bacterial infection called H. pylori (Helicobacter pylori). Over a long period of time, it can increase the risk of stomach cancer.

Not everyone infected with these viruses or bacteria will develop cancer.

Reducing your risk

You cannot protect yourself against all viruses and bacteria. But there are things you can do to reduce your risk of developing some of these:

HPV vaccination

Vaccines can be used to protect against HPV infection. The NHS offers the HPV vaccine to:

- girls from the age of 12 or 13
- boys from the age of 12 or 13.
- men who have sex with men.

Other people may also have the HPV vaccine, because they may have an increased risk of cancer caused by HPV infection. Your GP, local sexual health clinic or HIV clinic can give you more information.

Hepatitis B and C and HIV

Using condoms and dental dams during sex can help protect you from these.

If you inject drugs, it is important to never share needles. This is because viruses can pass from person to person in the blood.

Pre-cancerous conditions

Having a pre-cancerous condition does not mean that you have cancer, or that you will definitely develop cancer. But pre-cancerous conditions are diseases or syndromes that might develop into a cancer, so it's important to monitor your health.

1 October 2018

The above information is reprinted with kind permission from Macmillan Cancer Support.
© Macmillan Cancer Support 2023

www.macmillan.org.uk

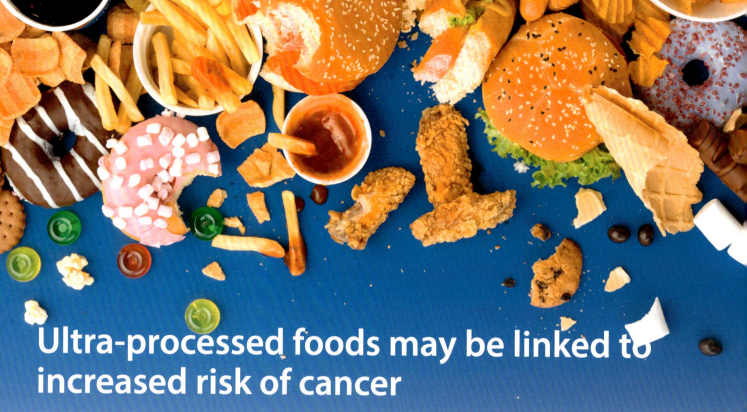

Ultra-processed foods may be linked to increased risk of cancer

Higher consumption of ultra-processed foods may be linked to an increased risk of developing and dying from cancer, an Imperial-led study suggests.

By Conrad Duncan

Researchers from Imperial's School of Public Health have produced the most comprehensive assessment to date of the association between ultra-processed foods and the risk of developing cancers. Ultra-processed foods are food items which have been heavily processed during their production, such as fizzy drinks, mass-produced packaged breads, many ready meals and most breakfast cereals.

Ultra-processed foods are often relatively cheap, convenient, and heavily marketed, often as healthy options. But these foods are also generally higher in salt, fat, sugar, and contain artificial additives. It is now well documented that they are linked with a range of poor health outcomes including obesity, type 2 diabetes and cardiovascular disease.

'This study adds to the growing evidence that ultra-processed foods are likely to negatively impact our health including our risk for cancer.'

– Dr Eszter Vamos, School of Public Health

The first UK study of its kind used UK Biobank records to collect information on the diets of 200,000 middle-aged adult participants. Researchers monitored participants' health over a 10-year period, looking at the risk of developing any cancer overall as well as the specific risk of developing 34 types of cancer. They also looked at the risk of people dying from cancer.

The study found that higher consumption of ultra-processed foods was associated with a greater risk of developing cancer overall, and specifically with ovarian and brain cancers. It was also associated with an increased risk of dying from cancer, most notably with ovarian and breast cancers.

For every 10 per cent increase in ultra-processed food in a person's diet, there was an increased incidence of 2 per cent for cancer overall, and a 19 per cent increase for ovarian cancer specifically.

Each 10 per cent increase in ultra-processed food consumption was also associated with increased mortality for cancer overall by 6 per cent, alongside a 16 per cent increase for breast cancer and a 30 per cent increase for ovarian cancer.

These links remained after adjusting for a range of socio-economic, behavioural and dietary factors, such as smoking status, physical activity and body mass index (BMI).

The Imperial team carried out the study, which is published in *eClinicalMedicine*, in collaboration with researchers from the International Agency for Research on Cancer (IARC), University of São Paulo, and NOVA University Lisbon.

Previous research from the team reported the levels of consumption of ultra-processed foods in the UK, which are the highest in Europe for both adults and children. The team also found that higher consumption of ultra-processed foods was associated with a greater risk of developing obesity and type 2 diabetes in UK adults, and a greater weight gain in UK children extending from childhood to young adulthood.

Dr Eszter Vamos, lead senior author for the study, from Imperial College London's School of Public Health, said: 'This study adds to the growing evidence that ultra-processed foods are likely to negatively impact our health including our risk for cancer. Given the high levels of consumption in UK adults and children, this has important implications for future health outcomes.

'Although our study cannot prove causation, other available evidence shows that reducing ultra-processed foods in our diet could provide important health benefits. Further research is needed to confirm these findings and understand the best public health strategies to reduce the widespread presence and harms of ultra-processed foods in our diet.'

> **'Our bodies may not react the same way to these ultra-processed ingredients and additives as they do to fresh and nutritious minimally processed foods.'**
>
> –Dr Kiara Chang, School of Public Health

Dr Kiara Chang, first author for the study, from Imperial College London's School of Public Health, said: 'The average person in the UK consumes more than half of their daily energy intake from ultra-processed foods. This is exceptionally high and concerning as ultra-processed foods are produced with industrially derived ingredients and often use food additives to adjust colour, flavour, consistency, texture, or extend shelf life.

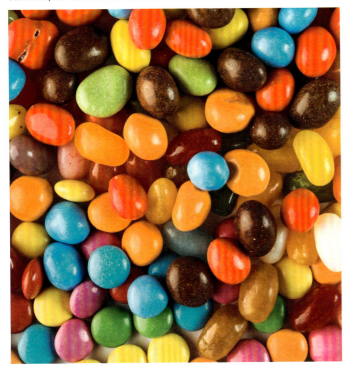

'Our bodies may not react the same way to these ultra-processed ingredients and additives as they do to fresh and nutritious minimally processed foods. However, ultra-processed foods are everywhere and highly marketed with cheap price and attractive packaging to promote consumption. This shows our food environment needs urgent reform to protect the population from ultra-processed foods.'

The World Health Organization and the United Nations' Food and Agriculture Organisation has previously recommended restricting ultra-processed foods as part of a healthy sustainable diet.

There are ongoing efforts to reduce ultra-processed food consumption around the world, with countries such as Brazil, France and Canada updating their national dietary guidelines with recommendations to limit such foods. Brazil has also banned the marketing of ultra-processed foods in schools. There are currently no similar measures to tackle ultra-processed foods in the UK.

Dr Chang added: 'We need clear front of pack warning labels for ultra-processed foods to aid consumer choices, and our sugar tax should be extended to cover ultra-processed fizzy drinks, fruit-based and milk-based drinks, as well as other ultra-processed products.

'Lower income households are particularly vulnerable to these cheap and unhealthy ultra-processed foods. Minimally processed and freshly prepared meals should be subsidised to ensure everyone has access to healthy, nutritious and affordable options.'

The researchers note that their study is observational, so does not show a causal link between ultra-processed foods and cancer due to the observational nature of the research. More work is needed in this area to establish a causal link.

1 February 2023

Mindmap

What are ultra-processed foods? Create a mindmap with different types of processed and ultra-processed foods.

Research

Do you eat ultra-processed food? Have a look at the ingredient list of one of the ultra-processed foods that you eat. How many ingredients do you recognise? Make a list of the unfamiliar ingredients and do some research on those ingredients and what their purpose is.

New genetic study confirms that alcohol is a direct cause of cancer

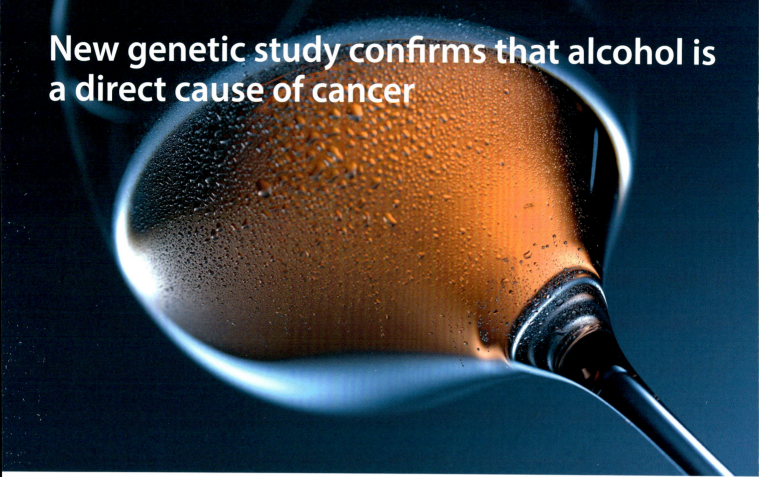

New data from a large-scale genetic study led by Oxford Population Health confirms that alcohol directly causes cancer.

Worldwide, alcohol may cause around 3 million deaths each year, including over 400,000 from cancer. With alcohol consumption rising, particularly in rapidly developing countries such as China, there is an urgent need to understand how alcohol affects disease risks in different populations.

Evidence from Western countries already strongly indicates that alcohol is a direct cause of cancer in the head, neck, oesophagus, liver, colon and breast. But it has been difficult to establish whether alcohol directly causes cancer, or if it is linked to possible confounding factors (such as smoking and diet) that could generate biased results. It was also unclear whether alcohol is linked to other types of cancer, including lung and stomach cancers.

To address these unknowns, researchers from Oxford Population Health, Peking University and the Chinese Academy of Medical Sciences, Beijing, used a genetic approach by investigating gene variants linked to lower alcohol consumption in Asian populations. The results have been published today in the International Journal of Cancer.

In Chinese, and other East Asian populations, two common genetic variants (alleles) reduce alcohol tolerability and are strongly associated with lower alcohol intake, because they cause an unpleasant 'flushing' effect. These mutations both disrupt the functioning of enzymes involved in alcohol detoxification, causing the toxic compound acetaldehyde, a Group I carcinogen, to accumulate in the blood.

The first mutation is a loss-of-function mutation in the gene for the enzyme aldehyde dehydrogenase 2 (ALDH2). The second mutation accelerates the activity of alcohol dehydrogenase 1B (ADH1B). Both are common in East Asians but rare in European ancestry populations.

Because these alleles are allocated at birth and are independent of other lifestyle factors (such as smoking), they can be used as a proxy for alcohol intake, to assess how alcohol consumption affects disease risks.

The study team used DNA samples from approximately 150,000 participants (roughly 60,000 men and 90,000 women) in the China Kadoorie Biobank study and measured the frequency of the low-alcohol tolerability alleles for ALDH2 and ADH1B. The data were combined with questionnaires about drinking habits completed by participants at recruitment and subsequent follow-up visits. The participants were tracked for a median period of 11 years through linkage to health insurance records and death registers.

Since women rarely drink alcohol in China, the main analysis focused on men, a third of whom drank regularly (most weeks in the past year).

Key results:

* Among the Chinese study population, the frequency of low-alcohol tolerability alleles was 21% for ALDH2 and

69% for ADH1B (compared with <0.01% and ~4% in European ancestry populations).

- In men, the low-alcohol tolerability alleles were strongly linked to reduced alcohol consumption, both frequency of drinking and mean alcohol intake.

- During the follow-up period, around 4,500 (7.4%) of the men developed cancer.

- Men carrying one or two of the low-alcohol tolerability alleles for ADH1B had between 13-25% lower risks of overall cancer and alcohol-related cancers, particularly head and neck cancer, and oesophageal cancer.

- Overall, men who carried two copies of the low-alcohol tolerability allele for ALDH2 drank very little alcohol, and had a 14% lower risk of developing any cancer, and a 31% lower risk of developing cancers that have previously been linked to alcohol (cancers of the head and neck; oesophagus, colon, rectum and liver).

Design

Design a poster with the dangers of drinking alcohol.

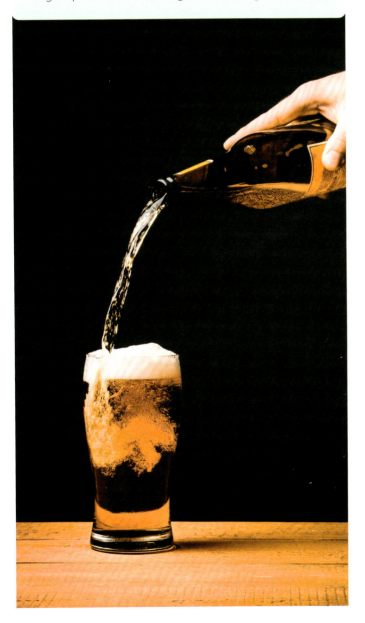

- Men who drank regularly despite carrying one copy of the low-alcohol tolerability allele for ALDH2 had significantly higher risks of head and neck cancer and oesophageal cancer. For non-drinkers or occasional drinkers, there was no overall association between carrying one copy of the low-alcohol tolerability allele for ALDH2 and increased cancer risk.

The results remained the same when the data were adjusted for other cancer risk factors, such as smoking, diet, physical activity, body mass and family history of cancer.

In women (only 2% of whom drank regularly), these low-alcohol tolerability alleles were not associated with any increased risk of cancer, indicating that the reduced risks for the carriers of these gene variants in men directly resulted from their lower alcohol consumption.

The significantly greater risks seen in men carrying the low-alcohol tolerability ALDH2 gene variant who still drank regularly suggests that greater accumulation of acetaldehyde may directly increase cancer risk.

Lead researcher Dr Pek Kei (Becky) Im from Oxford Population Health said: 'These findings indicate that alcohol directly causes several types of cancer, and that these risks may be increased further in people with inherited low alcohol tolerability who cannot properly metabolise alcohol.'

Senior researcher Dr Iona Millwood from Oxford Population Health said: 'Our study reinforces the need to lower population levels of alcohol consumption for cancer prevention, especially in China where alcohol consumption is increasing despite the low alcohol tolerability among a large subset of the population.'

20 January 2022

Read & Write

How did the researchers confirm that alcohol is a direct cause of cancer?

Pick out some key sentences and write a paragraph describing how the researchers confirmed their theory.

How does smoking cause cancer?

- Smoking is the biggest preventable cause of cancer in the UK, and worldwide.

- Harmful chemicals in cigarette smoke affect the entire body – not just our lungs. And smoking causes at least 15 different cancer types.

- There is no safe level of smoking – stopping completely is the best thing you can do for your health, and there are many support and quitting options available.

What's my cancer risk from smoking?

Our bodies are designed to deal with a bit of damage, but they often can't cope with the amount of harmful chemicals in tobacco smoke.

Both the amount you smoke, and the length of time you've been smoking for affect your cancer risk.

The more cigarettes you smoke a day, the higher your risk of cancer, so reducing the number of daily cigarettes you smoke can be a good first step.

But the number of years you spend smoking affects your cancer risk most strongly. So it's important to make a plan to stop smoking completely.

Remember, the sooner you stop, the lower your risk of cancer. Everyone who smokes can benefit from stopping, and it's never too late to stop – even if you've smoked for years.

Speak to your GP or pharmacist, or visit NHS Smokefree for free support to help you stop for good.

Smoking, DNA damage and cancer

DNA is found in all our cells and controls how they behave. Even one cigarette can damage DNA.

1. Cigarette smoke releases over 5000 chemicals and many of these are harmful – we know at least 70 can cause cancer.

2. The harmful chemicals enter our lungs and spread around the entire body.

3. Chemicals from cigarettes damage DNA.

4. Cigarette chemicals make it harder for cells to repair any DNA damage. They also damage the parts of DNA that protect us from cancer.

5. It's the build-up of DNA damage in the same cell over time that leads to cancer.

Smoking is the leading cause of lung cancer

Smoking causes more than 7 in 10 lung cancer cases in the UK. Lung cancer is the most common cause of cancer death.

People who smoke sometimes have a cough. But coughing can also be a sign of lung cancer, as well as other conditions. So if you have any doubt, or a cough or other symptom that's new, changing, or won't go away, talk to your doctor.

How can smoking cause cancer?

1 Cigarette smoke releases over 5,000 different chemicals

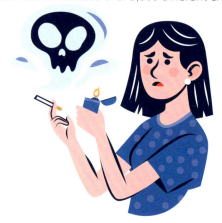

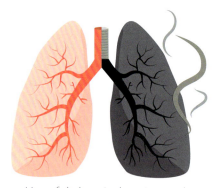

2 Harmful chemicals enter our lungs and then affect the entire body

3 Chemicals damage our DNA, including parts that protect us from cancer

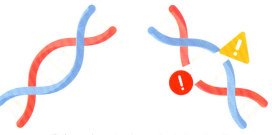

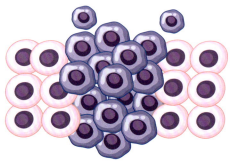

4 Other chemicals make it harder for cells to repair DNA damage

5 This DNA damage can cause cancer in cells

Source: Cancer Research UK

Being smoke free can prevent 15 types of cancer

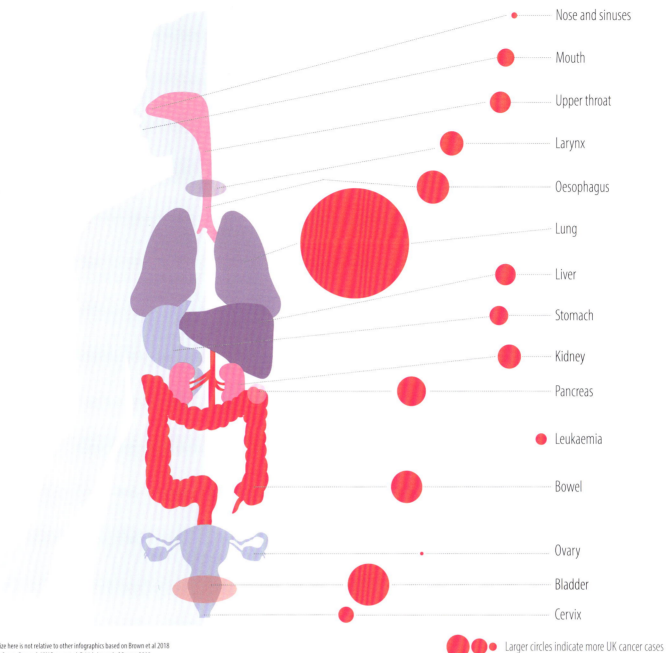

- Nose and sinuses
- Mouth
- Upper throat
- Larynx
- Oesophagus
- Lung
- Liver
- Stomach
- Kidney
- Pancreas
- Leukaemia
- Bowel
- Ovary
- Bladder
- Cervix

Circle size here is not relative to other infographics based on Brown et al 2018
Source: Cancer Research UK/ Brown et al, British Journal of Cancer, 2018

Larger circles indicate more UK cancer cases

And remember it's never too late to stop smoking and reduce your lung cancer risk. The best way to reduce your risk is to stop smoking completely. Have a read of our tips and support to help you quit smoking for good.

What other types of cancer does smoking cause?

The link between smoking and cancer is very clear. It causes at least 15 different types of cancer, including two of the most common, lung and bowel cancer.

Other cancers caused by smoking include mouth, pharynx (upper throat), nose and sinuses, larynx (voice box), oesophagus (food pipe), liver, pancreas, stomach, kidney, ovary, bladder, cervix, and some types of leukaemia.

Smoking causes other diseases too, such as heart disease and various lung diseases.

Light, occasional and social smoking also cause cancer

There is no safe level of smoking.

Smoking 1-10 cigarettes per day increases the risk of getting smoking-related cancers and other diseases.

Even smoking less than one cigarette per day is harmful. One study found that it significantly increases the risk of dying early compared with people who have never smoked.

The best thing you can do for your health is to stop smoking completely.

19 March 2021

Cancer in children and young people – what do the statistics tell us?

1. Every day in the UK 10 children or young people are diagnosed with cancer

While cancer is rare in children and young people, there are around 3,755 young people diagnosed with cancer each year in the UK. That's 1,645 in children (aged 0-14 years) and 2,110 in teenagers and young adults (aged 15-24 years).

Cancer is more common in young males. Around 1 in every 420 boys under the age of 15 developed cancer compared to 1 in 490 girls. For young people aged 15-24, it was 1 in every 360 for males and 1 in 380 for females.

For both males and females, cancer incidence is higher in the first five years of life, falls to its lowest rate at age 5 to 9 years, and then starts to increase again from 10 years of age marking the start of an unbroken rise in incidence that continues into the teenage years and throughout adulthood.

The most common cancers diagnosed in children aged 0-14 years in the UK, based on cancers registered between 1997 and 2016

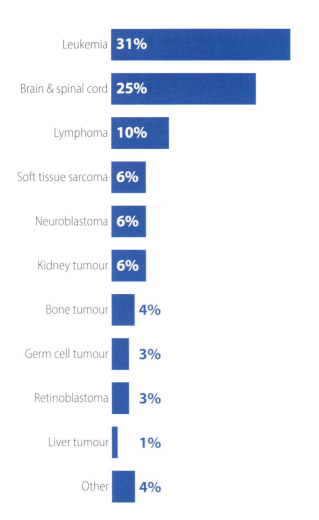

Leukemia — 31%
Brain & spinal cord — 25%
Lymphoma — 10%
Soft tissue sarcoma — 6%
Neuroblastoma — 6%
Kidney tumour — 6%
Bone tumour — 4%
Germ cell tumour — 3%
Retinoblastoma — 3%
Liver tumour — 1%
Other — 4%

Source: National Cancer Registration and Analysis Service for England (Public Health England), the Northern Ireland Cancer Registry, the Scottish Cancer Registry, and the Welsh Cancer Intelligence and Surveillance Unit

The most common cancers diagnosed in teenagers and young adults aged 15-24 years in the UK, based on cancers registered between 1997 and 2016

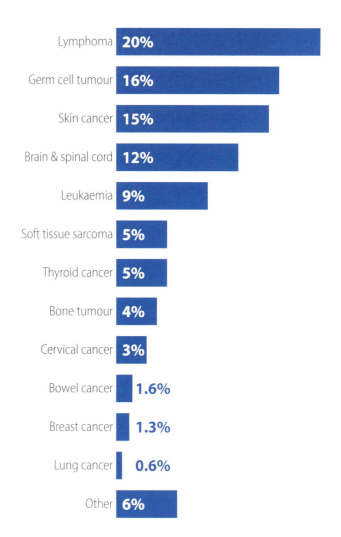

Lymphoma — 20%
Germ cell tumour — 16%
Skin cancer — 15%
Brain & spinal cord — 12%
Leukaemia — 9%
Soft tissue sarcoma — 5%
Thyroid cancer — 5%
Bone tumour — 4%
Cervical cancer — 3%
Bowel cancer — 1.6%
Breast cancer — 1.3%
Lung cancer — 0.6%
Other — 6%

Source: National Cancer Registration and Analysis Service for England (Public Health England), the Northern Ireland Cancer Registry, the Scottish Cancer Registry, and the Welsh Cancer Intelligence and Surveillance Unit

2. Children and young people get different types of cancer compared to adults

Children and young people get different types of cancer to adults and are generally more treatable.

The most common cancers for adults are lung, breast and bowel cancers. The most common type of cancer in children is leukaemia, which accounts for about a third of all cases in this age group. A further quarter of cancer cases are brain and spinal cord tumours. 1 in 10 are lymphomas.

For young people aged 15-24, 1 in 5 of cases are lymphomas. Around 1 in 6 are germ cell tumours, most of which are testicular cancers. Around 1 in 7 are skin cancers, 1 in 8 are brain and spinal cord tumours and 1 in 11 are leukaemia.

Five year survival of children, teenagers and young adults aged 0-24 years with cancer in the UK

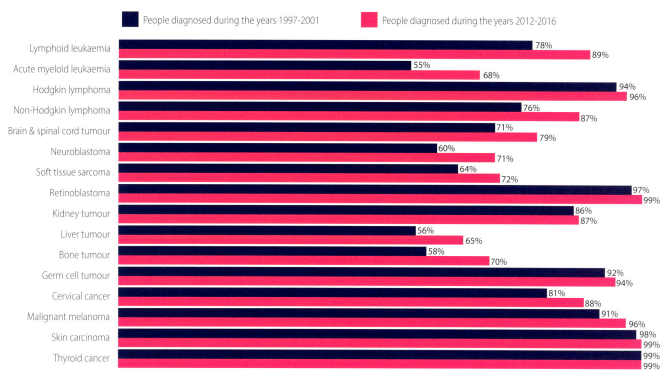

Legend: People diagnosed during the years 1997-2001 (navy) / People diagnosed during the years 2012-2016 (pink)

Cancer type	1997-2001	2012-2016
Lymphoid leukaemia	78%	89%
Acute myeloid leukaemia	55%	68%
Hodgkin lymphoma	94%	96%
Non-Hodgkin lymphoma	76%	87%
Brain & spinal cord tumour	71%	79%
Neuroblastoma	60%	71%
Soft tissue sarcoma	64%	72%
Retinoblastoma	97%	99%
Kidney tumour	86%	87%
Liver tumour	56%	65%
Bone tumour	58%	70%
Germ cell tumour	92%	94%
Cervical cancer	81%	88%
Malignant melanoma	91%	96%
Skin carcinoma	98%	99%
Thyroid cancer	99%	99%

Based on observed survival. Source: National Cancer Registration and Analysis Service for England (Public Health England), the Northern Ireland Cancer Registry, the Scottish Cancer Registry, and the Welsh Cancer Intelligence and Surveillance Unit

3. Around 1 in 5 cancers diagnosed in teenagers and young adults may be preventable

Around 15% of cancers diagnosed in people aged 15-24 years are skin cancers, which may be preventable by avoiding UV light exposure and burns from sunlight and use of sunbeds.

Cervical cancer accounts for 6% of cancers in females aged 15-24 and is largely preventable by the vaccination against human papillomavirus (HPV).

4. Cancer survival in children and young people has improved for most cancers

More than eight out of ten young people diagnosed with cancer survive at least five years, and many of these are cured. Thanks to research and better treatment, survival has increased over the past 20 years.

Overall, 78% of children and young people diagnosed in 1997 to 2001 survived for at least five years. This went up to 86% for those diagnosed in 2012 to 2016: a statistically significant increase.

There was a marked increase in survival between these periods for children and young people with leukaemia, lymphomas, brain and spinal cord tumours, bone tumours, soft tissue sarcomas, neuroblastoma and malignant melanomas.

The highest survival rates were for Hodgkin lymphoma, retinoblastoma, germ cell tumours, and skin and thyroid cancers, with over 90% surviving five years after diagnosis.

There are several cancers that have poorer survival that need further research and better treatments, notably some of the brain cancers, bone tumours and soft tissue sarcomas.

5. Our data helps the understanding of children's and young people's cancers

Robust data gathering and analysis is a major part of what population-based cancer registries do. Reliable data on cancer incidence and survival across the population is important for understanding all cancers, including cancer in children and young people.

This information is essential for clinicians, health services and policy makers as it helps them work out what resources are needed to improve the care, diagnosis and treatment of cancer in children and young people.

This information helps children and young people with cancer, their families, and charities, understand more about the disease. This knowledge can make a real difference when dealing with something that is so emotionally challenging.

These data also help researchers compare on a global scale how the UK is performing compared to other countries.

This study is based in part on information collected and quality assured by the National Cancer Registration and Analysis Service (part of Public Health England), the Northern Ireland Cancer Registry, the Welsh Cancer Intelligence and Surveillance Unit (part of Public Health Wales) and the Scottish Cancer Registry (Public Health Scotland).

This work uses data provided by patients and collected by health services as part of their care and support.

15 March 2021

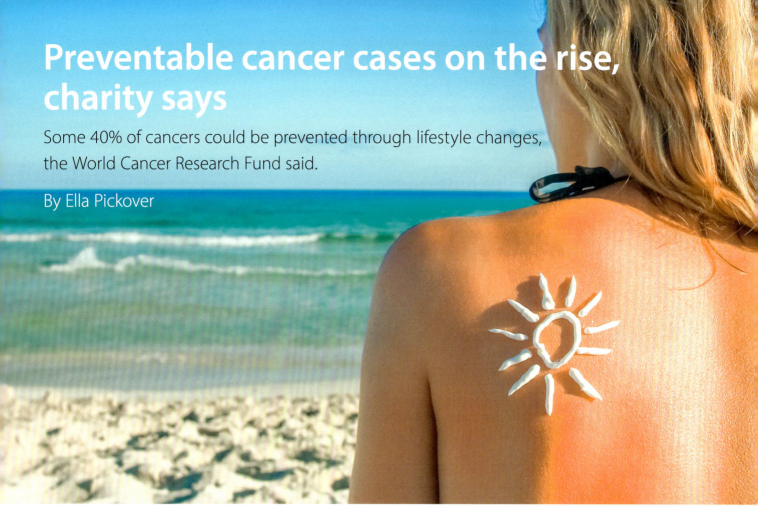

Preventable cancer cases on the rise, charity says

Some 40% of cancers could be prevented through lifestyle changes, the World Cancer Research Fund said.

By Ella Pickover

Drinking, tanning and smoking are contributing to around 400 'preventable' cases of cancer every day in the UK, new estimates have suggested.

The World Cancer Research Fund (WCRF) has estimated that about 155,000 cases of cancer could be prevented every year if people led different lifestyles.

It said that some 387,820 people were diagnosed with cancer in 2019/20, the latest figures available.

However, people leading unhealthy lifestyles mean this figure is higher than it should be.

The charity said that, compared with 2017 data, there was an increase of 8,000 'preventable cases'.

It said that about 40% of cancers could be prevented through lifestyle changes such as eating healthily, being active, maintaining a healthy weight and not smoking.

> **'Screening plays a vital role in improving cancer outcomes – the earlier someone is diagnosed, the more likely they are to survive'**
> –Vanessa Gordon-Dseagu, WCRF

People can also stop drinking alcohol, cut back their red meat consumption and avoid processed meat to help reduce their risk of cancer.

They can also stay safe in the sun and breastfeed where possible, the charity added.

'Over the years, research has estimated that around 40% of cancers are associated with modifiable risk factors,' said Dr Vanessa Gordon-Dseagu, research interpretation manager at WCRF.

'These risk factors include smoking and limiting sun exposure.

'Alongside this, research has shown that, by following WCRF's cancer prevention recommendations, individuals can reduce their cancer risk.

'It is also important to remember that our population is ageing, so we are likely to see incidence of cancer continue to increase over the next few decades.

'Screening plays a vital role in improving cancer outcomes – the earlier someone is diagnosed, the more likely they are to survive.'

It comes after Cancer Research UK said that 'ending smoking' would slash the number of cancer cases which are linked to deprivation.

A study published last week in the journal PLOS One found that if nobody in England smoked then cancer cases linked to deprivation would reduce from 27,200 to 16,500.

27 September 2022

What's the story behind the new UK cancer statistics?

By Rob Mansfield

Cancer incidence, mortality and survival data from across the devolved nations (England, Wales, Scotland and Northern Ireland) are routinely collected via cancer registries. Globally, UK cancer data is considered among the most accurate and, while this data may be updated throughout the year, new datasets are usually released only once a year.

What do the UK cancer statistics tell us?

Our team at World Cancer Research Fund has collated the latest cancer data available from the devolved nations to give us an overall UK-wide set of cancer statistics. The figures are from 2019 and 2020, and include new incidence and mortality data.

They show that in the UK, 387,820 people were diagnosed with cancer and 166,502 people died from cancer during these years, an increase from 366,303 and 165,267, respectively, from 2017.

Breast, followed by lung, cancer remains most common in the UK. Overall, there were more cancer cases in men than in women.

We're all getting older

One reason for the increase in cases is that in recent decades we've seen an increase in life expectancy. Age is the most important risk factor for cancer so as life expectancy increases, so too will the number of people diagnosed with cancer.

However, in the last few years, life expectancy in the UK and other industrialised nations has declined. In the coming years, it will be important for us to understand the factors that are influencing these declines in life expectancy.

At World Cancer Research Fund we'll be working across our research and policy areas to understand the data and play our part to improve life expectancy and cancer outcomes.

Prostate cancer on the rise

There's been a noticeable increase in diagnoses of prostate cancer in the past few years. Comparing 2017 data with 2019 data, we can see that recorded cases of prostate cancer have seen an increase of over 13%.

Why are we seeing this increase and is it because we're becoming less healthy? Not necessarily – the charity Prostate Cancer UK says it's likely that more men are getting tested, possibly inspired by celebrities sharing their own prostate cancer journeys: Stephen Fry revealed his prostate cancer diagnosis in 2018 and Bill Turnbull sadly died of the disease this month.

This partially explains why prostate cancer is the 2nd most common cancer in the UK, yet sits slightly lower worldwide in 4th position.

Lung cancer curbed by tobacco control

Lung cancer is still the 3rd most common cancer in the UK and accounted for 20% of cancer deaths. However, the number of cases in the UK decreased between the 2017 and 2019/2020 data – a trend that has been seen since the 1990s. This reflects the declining rates of smoking in the past 10 years brought about by strong tobacco control measures.

The picture in the UK contrasts with the global one – where lung cancer cases rose between 2018 and 2020.

Increase in cancer cases

The fact that nearly all cancer types have seen an increase in cases does, however, strengthen the importance of cancer prevention. We know that around 40% of cancers could be prevented, that's 155,000 cancer cases a year, if everyone followed our Cancer Prevention Recommendations – including eating healthily, being active, maintaining a healthy weight and not drinking alcohol, as well as avoiding smoking and sun exposure.

Other ways include eating no more than 3 portions of red meat a week and little, if any, processed meat, and new mothers breastfeeding if you can – which is good for mothers and babies.

Let's take bowel cancer, for example. Our research shows that a poor diet – high in processed meat and low in fibre and vegetables – coupled with obesity, a lack of physical activity and drinking alcohol increases an individual's risk of developing the disease.

In 2019, cases of bowel cancer rose by nearly 3%, from 2017 data, to close to 45,000 people. What a difference it would make if people started following our Cancer Prevention Recommendations more closely.

27 September 2022

www.wcrf-uk.org

Global melanoma rate to increase by 50% by 2040, researchers predict

Australia's skin cancer rate rising in over 50s, but 'declining quite steeply' among younger age groups.

By Donna Lu

New cases of melanoma are set to increase by 50% globally by 2040, with a 68% increase in deaths, according to new research.

An international team of researchers have analysed the global burden of melanoma, which accounts for approximately one in five skin cancers. Data from the International Agency for Research on Cancer estimated that there were 325,000 new melanoma cases and 57,000 deaths in 2020.

The study, published in the journal JAMA Dermatology, found the cumulative risk of developing melanoma was highest in Australia and New Zealand, where one in 20 men and one in 30 women were affected by 75 years of age.

The estimated incidence – the number of new cases in a given period – was 36 times greater in Australia than in many African and Asian countries, while the highest death rates from the skin cancer were seen in New Zealand.

'Essentially that is because of our largely fair-skinned populations living in countries where we have very high ultraviolet radiation,' said study co-author Prof Anne Cust, of Melanoma Institute Australia.

Cust, also deputy director of the Daffodil Centre, said the paper 'highlights how important it is to make some changes so that we can reduce the impact of melanoma.'

Melanoma Institute Australia last month released a report calling for long-term investment in a national melanoma prevention and awareness campaign.

Based on the incidence of melanoma in 2020, the study's authors estimated that the health burden of cancer will increase to 510,000 new cases and 96,000 deaths globally by 2040.

The projected rise in the number of people dying from melanoma in coming decades was largely driven by ageing populations, said study co-author Prof David Whiteman, an epidemiologist at the QIMR Berghofer Medical Research Institute.

In Australia, rates of melanoma have plateaued in recent years, but differ starkly among age groups, Whiteman said. Rates of melanoma were continuing to rise in people in their 50s and older, he said, while for 'people in their 20s, 30s and 40s, rates are actually declining quite steeply'.

'The most likely explanation is that the older people are still paying the price for sun exposure they incurred maybe decades ago, before Slip-Slop-Slap,' Whiteman said.

Researchers are still learning more about skin cancer differences between men and woman. 'Women have high rates of melanoma … before age of 50, in most countries in the world,' Whiteman said. 'Then after 50, men's rates tend to really take off.'

While women are more likely to get melanomas on their legs, men tend to get them on their back, head and neck, said Whiteman. 'That is a consistent observation around populations around the world.' The discrepancies were most likely due to differing patterns of sun exposure, he said.

Chair of Cancer Council's national skin cancer committee, Heather Walker, who was not involved in the study, said the findings were not surprising but highlighted the need for sustained awareness and prevention campaigns. 'Given melanoma is such a preventable cancer, we could do more globally to improve prevention messages,' she said.

'We're spending $1.7bn a year on treating all types of skin cancer in Australia. That's the highest amount of spend on any cancer type,' Walker said. 'Investment in prevention is very modest by comparison.

'Not only are there health gains but there are also financial gains to be made in investing in prevention.'

Cust agreed. 'We do have a new campaign that's just starting with two years of funding, but we're really looking for more ongoing sustained funding.'

'When you introduce a new prevention campaign, you don't see the results of that the next year. Cancers take a long time to develop – you see the impact of that in 10 years' time, 20 years' time.

'It's really important that people do take preventive actions. We know, for example, that wearing sunscreen reduces risk even at older ages. Even if you've had sun damage in the past, it's important to use preventive behaviours.'

30 March 2022

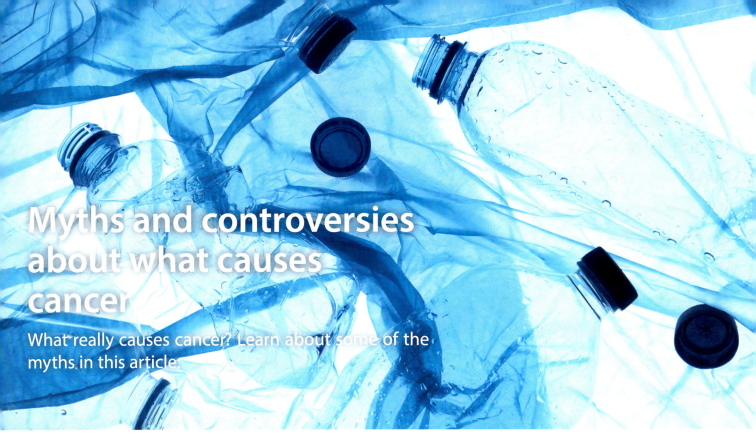

Myths and controversies about what causes cancer

What really causes cancer? Learn about some of the myths in this article.

O ur health information team explore what other organisations are saying about the rumours, fiction, media reports and urban legends about whether everyday products increase cancer risk.

Vegan diets

Following a vegan diet means only eating plant-based foods and avoiding all animal products including meat, dairy and eggs.

There is no direct evidence that following a vegan diet reduces the risk of developing cancer. However, there are many characteristics of a healthy vegan diet that align with our Cancer Prevention Recommendations – such as eating lots of wholegrains, pulses, fruit and vegetables, and avoiding red and processed meat.

This is not only because plant-based foods contain fibre, which protects against bowel cancer, but including more plant-based food in the diet can also help people to maintain a healthy weight – and being overweight or obese increases the risk of 12 types of cancer.

We also know that eating red and processed meat increases the risk of bowel cancer. There is no evidence to suggest consuming white meat or fish increases the risk of cancer.

Plastic bottles and cling film

There are claims that chemicals in plastic drinks bottles, cling film and food containers can cause cancer by seeping into the contents. While some studies have shown that a very small amount of chemicals in plastic packaging can get into drinks or food when heated, these amounts have been well within safe limits – which are very strictly regulated in the UK.

There is no reliable evidence that using plastic bottles to drink from, or cling film to store or freeze food, increases your risk of cancer. However, if you are using plastic utensils while cooking, the best thing to do is to follow the directions and only use plastics that are specifically meant for cooking. Inert containers, such as heat-resistant glass, ceramics and stainless steel, are preferable for cooking.

The risk of using plastics for cooking is very small. Not smoking, followed by maintaining a healthy weight through eating a healthy diet and keeping active, are the most effective ways to reduce your cancer risk.

Artificial sweeteners

Studies on artificial sweeteners, including saccharin and aspartame, have shown no convincing evidence of an association with cancer. Earlier cancer scares linked with certain sweeteners have been discredited.

Not smoking, followed by maintaining a healthy weight through eating a healthy diet and keeping active, are the most effective ways to reduce your cancer risk.

Psychological stress

Some people have suggested a link between psychological stress (which is what people experience when under mental, physical or emotional pressure) and an increased risk of cancer. However, there is no strong evidence for this. Most studies have not found that such stress increases the risk of cancer.

However, people under stress can sometimes behave in unhealthy ways, such as smoking, overeating or drinking heavily, which do increase their risk of many cancers. If you're under stress, it's important to try to find other ways of coping, such as doing physical activity.

Cosmetics and toiletries

Most studies have found no link between cancer and the chemicals used in cosmetic and toiletry products such as moisturisers, shampoos, deodorants, and toothpastes. The majority of countries have strict regulations to ensure these products are safe.

Some studies have found a link between talcum powder (talc) and ovarian cancer, but there is not enough evidence to be certain of this. Even if there were an increased risk, scientists estimate it would be small. Not smoking, followed by maintaining a healthy weight through eating a healthy diet and keeping active, are the most effective ways to reduce your cancer risk.

Breast implants

There have been many studies into whether silicone leakage from breast implants increases the risk of breast cancer. None of them so far have found any evidence that this is the case. Not smoking, followed by maintaining a healthy weight through eating a healthy diet and keeping active, are the most effective ways to reduce your cancer risk.

Underwire bras

The majority of research has found no link between the use of underwire bras and breast cancer. Not smoking, followed by maintaining a healthy weight through eating a healthy diet and keeping active, are the most effective ways to reduce your cancer risk.

Organic food

Organic farming makes use of crop rotation, environmental management and good animal husbandry to control pests and diseases. This means that there are limited additives used in organic food production. Processed organic foods use ingredients that are produced organically, and for a food to be certified organic, at least 95% of the food must be made up of organic ingredients.

There are many different reasons why consumers choose to buy organic food, such as concern for the environment and animal welfare. Consumers may also choose to buy organic food because they believe it is safer and more nutritious than other food and that artificial fertilisers and pesticides may increase the risk of some diseases, including cancer.

Two large studies have looked at organic food consumption and cancer risk. The Million Women Study, a large study of UK women, showed in 2014 little or no decrease in the incidence of cancer associated with consumption of organic food.

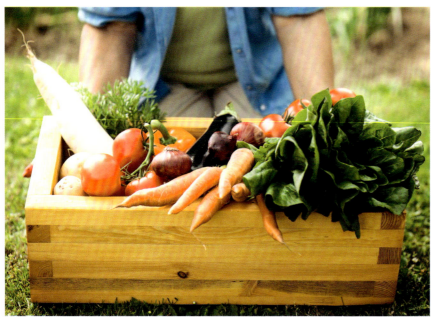

A study published in 2018 in a large group of French adults showed that people who had more organic foods, more often, in their diets had a lower risk of several types of cancer.

However, this is a single study and due to its design, it is not possible to be sure that the organic food was causing the lower risk of cancer. There may be other factors, such as income, which influence the results.

There is currently limited evidence to suggest that organic foods may offer added protection against cancer compared to conventionally grown produce.

Research shows that eating a healthy diet, along with not smoking and keeping active, are very important in cancer prevention, but choosing fresh, frozen, canned, conventional or organic produce does not affect your cancer risk.

Pesticides

Both organic and conventional food have to meet the same legal food safety requirements. Before pesticides are approved they are rigorously assessed to ensure they do not pose an unacceptable risk to human health or the environment, and that any pesticide residues left in food will not be harmful to consumers.

Pesticide residues in the food chain are also monitored to check they are within legal and safe limits. Additives are also subject to rigorous, pre-market safety assessments before they can be used in foods. Their use is controlled by legal limits, which ensures consumption does not exceed safe levels.

Hormones in cattle

Legislation about hormones in cattle varies from country to country. For example, growth hormones are used in dairy farming in the US, whereas the use of hormonal growth promoters for livestock is banned in the UK. Antibiotic growth-promoting feed additives have also been phased out due to concerns about the potential spread of antibiotic resistance.

Bovine somatotropin (or BST) is a hormone used to increase milk or meat production in cattle and is banned in the UK and Europe but is licensed in the US. BST was banned on animal welfare grounds, not because there is any proven effect on human health. An EU Scientific Committee report has stated that there is no scientific evidence that this hormone is a health risk.

Milk is rigorously tested for traces of antibiotics by law to ensure that food is safe for consumption. Cows receiving antibiotics are milked separately from the rest of the herd to ensure that the milk is discarded and does not enter the food supply.

In the UK, the Food Standards Agency regulates the content of milk and other dairy products to ensure these products are safe to consume.

Not smoking, followed by maintaining a healthy weight through eating a healthy diet and keeping active, are the most effective ways to reduce your cancer risk. Research

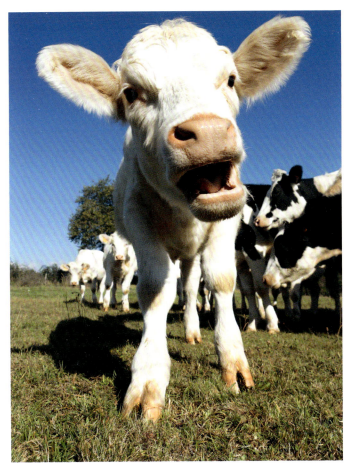

For general health, research from the European Food Safety Authority (EFSA) shows it is safe for healthy adults, including pregnant women, to drink single doses of up to 200mg of caffeine. Drinking up to 400mg of caffeine through the day does not raise safety concerns in the general population, which is equal to around four cups of filter coffee a day.

Burnt or browned foods (Acrylamide)

The UK's Food Standards Agency has recommended that foods with a high starch content, such as bread, chips and potatoes, should be cooked to a golden yellow colour, rather than brown, to reduce intake of a chemical that has been associated with causing cancer in mice.

Acrylamide is present in many different types of food and is a natural by-product of the cooking process. The highest levels of the substance are found in foods with high-starch content which have been cooked above 120C, such as crisps, bread, breakfast cereals, biscuits, crackers, cakes and coffee (as a result of the roasted beans).

It can also be produced during home cooking, when high-starch foods – such as potatoes, chips, bread and parsnips – are baked, roasted, grilled or fried at high temperatures. When bread is grilled to make toast, for example, this causes more acrylamide to be produced. The darker the colour of the toast, the more acrylamide is present.

However, the research linking acrylamide to cancer has only been carried out using animals. The World Cancer Research Fund has carried out a review of studies in people, and found no link between acrylamide in food and cancer. More research is needed but, in the meantime, maintaining a healthy weight and eating a healthy diet – together with not smoking and keeping active, are the most effective ways to reduce your cancer risk.

shows that eating too much red meat, and any amount of processed meat, increases the risk of bowel cancer. For cancer prevention, it is best to eat no more than about three portions a week of red meat (350 to 500 grams in total cooked weight), such as beef, pork and lamb, and to eat little, if any, processed meat, such as ham and bacon.

Food additives

Food additives are ingredients added to foods for various reasons – for example, to add colour, enhance flavours or to make them last longer. All additives, including artificial sweeteners, are assessed for safety before they are used in foods. An E number is a reference number given to food additives that have passed safety tests and have been approved for use in the UK and throughout the European Union.

The only additives for which evidence has shown a link with cancer are nitrites and nitrates, which are used as preservatives in processed meat. Eating processed meat is strongly associated with an increased risk of bowel cancer.

There is currently no other strong evidence linking food additives to an increased cancer risk.

Coffee

There is no strong evidence that coffee increases cancer risk, but there is strong evidence that coffee can actually reduce the risk of womb (endometrial) and liver cancer. However, we cannot make any specific recommendations because there are too many unanswered questions – for example, are the benefits a result of drinking coffee regularly, or in large amounts? There is also no evidence on the effects of adding milk and/or sugar, or on drinking caffeinated, decaffeinated, instant or filter coffee.

Tap water

WCRF research has found that drinking water contaminated with arsenic increases the risk of skin, lung and bladder cancer. Water contaminated with arsenic is not a public health issue in the UK, although it does affect some other countries that have high natural concentrations of arsenic in soil.

In some parts of the UK, fluoride is added to the water supply to help prevent tooth decay. Public Health England monitors the effects of water fluoridation on health. To date, there is no evidence of a difference in the rate for all types of cancer between fluoridated and non-fluoridated areas.

Water is a healthier choice than many other drinks, particularly compared with those high in sugar and calories, which can contribute to weight gain. Not smoking, followed by maintaining a healthy weight through eating a healthy diet and keeping active, are the most effective ways to reduce your cancer risk.

The above information is reprinted with kind permission from World Cancer Research Fund UK.
© 2023 World Cancer Research Fund UK

www.wcrf-uk.org

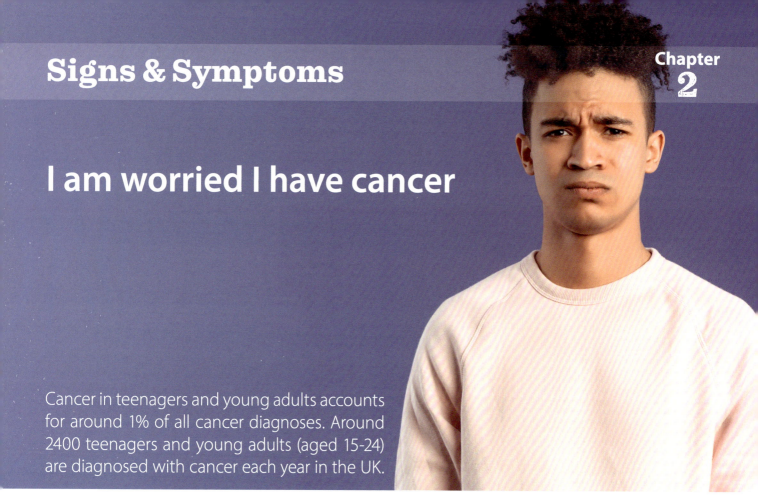

I am worried I have cancer

Cancer in teenagers and young adults accounts for around 1% of all cancer diagnoses. Around 2400 teenagers and young adults (aged 15-24) are diagnosed with cancer each year in the UK.

If you are worried about any changes in your body, it's important to get these checked out by your GP. If you have any of the symptoms below, especially if they last for a while or you can't explain them, you should make an appointment with your doctor.

Common symptoms

- Pain, that doesn't go away quickly when you take painkillers

- A lump or swelling anywhere on your body

- Unexplained weight loss

- Tiredness

- Headaches or dizziness that won't go away

- Changes to moles - for example changes in size or colour, or if they start bleeding

- Changes to bowel habits (going to the toilet) that last for more than a few weeks

- Unexplained bruising

- Breathlessness

- Symptoms that refuse to clear up, e.g. a cough or hoarseness that last for more than three weeks

- Sweating a lot at night

- Unexplained bleeding - for example coughing up blood, blood in your urine or poo, bleeding after sex, between periods or blood in your vomit if you are sick.

Common cancers

The most common cancer in young men aged 15-24 is testicular cancer, followed by Hodgkin's lymphoma and leukaemia. The most common cancers in young women aged 15-24 are melanoma, Hodgkin's lymphoma and ovarian cancer.

Testicular cancer

The most common symptoms of testicular cancer are:

- a lump in the testicle

- pain or discomfort

- a heavy scrotum

Melanoma

The most common symptoms of melanoma are a mole that is:

- getting bigger

- changing shape, particularly getting an irregular edge

- changing colour - getting darker, becoming patchy or having different colours

- painful or itching

- bleeding or becoming crusty

- looking inflamed

Hodgkin lymphoma

The most common symptoms of Hodgkin lymphoma are:

- swelling in the neck, armpit or groin, that is usually painless

- heavy sweating, especially at night

- losing a lot of weight over a short period of time

- high temperatures that come and go, often overnight, and with no obvious cause

- itching, which may feel worse after drinking alcohol

- coughing or breathlessness

- abdominal pain or vomiting after drinking alcohol

Ovarian cancer

The most common symptoms of ovarian cancer include:

- pain in the lower abdomen or side

- bloated, full feeling in the abdomen

- abdominal pain

- back pain

- passing urine more often than usual

- constipation

- pain during sex

- a swollen abdomen

- loss of appetite

- irregular periods or unexplained vaginal bleeding

Brain tumours

Brain tumours can be particularly hard to diagnose and can cause a number of different symptoms. A routine eye test by an optician can sometimes detect warning signs of pressure build-up at the back of the eye as a result of a brain tumour.

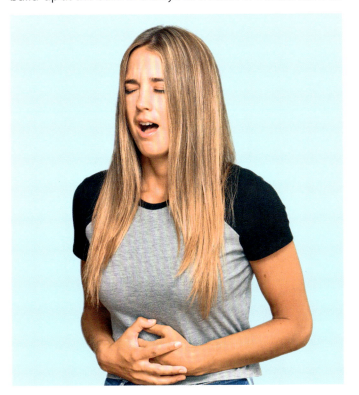

Signs and symptoms of brain tumours include:

- Persistent or recurrent vomiting

- Persistent or recurrent headache

- Abnormal eye movements

- Blurred or double vision, or loss of vision

- Balance/coordination/walking problems

- Behaviour change

- Fits or seizures

- Delayed puberty

If you have any signs or symptoms that might be cancer, it's important to make an appointment with your GP as soon as possible. Your appointment might be in-person or over the phone/by video call.

- If it turns out not to be cancer, you haven't wasted anyone's time. You'll still be listened to and taken seriously.

- If it does turn out to be cancer, then getting diagnosed early is really important, as early treatment will improve the outcome.

It's normal to feel nervous about speaking to your doctor. It can help to:

- Write down what you want to say and ask beforehand

- Make a note of your symptoms and when you started to feel unwell

- Share as much information as possible – little details can make a big difference

- Take a friend or someone from your family with you

- Be open and honest – remember that doctors talk to people about all kinds of problems all day, every day

- Ask your doctor to repeat anything you don't understand

- Make sure you know what will happen next before you leave

Getting diagnosed with cancer

Diagnosis means finding out whether you have cancer and, if so, what type of cancer you have. Doctors will do this by assessing you, and your symptoms, and by doing tests.

If you have symptoms that could be caused by cancer, you will be referred by your GP or local hospital to a specialist doctor in teenager and young adult cancer.

13 cancer symptoms you should get checked now

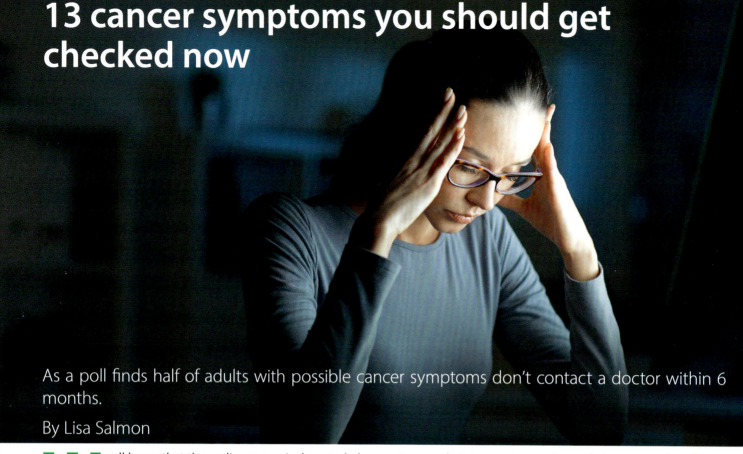

As a poll finds half of adults with possible cancer symptoms don't contact a doctor within 6 months.

By Lisa Salmon

We all know that the earlier cancer is detected, the better the chance of survival. Yet new research has found half of UK adults with a possible cancer symptom don't contact their GP within six months.

A YouGov poll of 2,468 people for Cancer Research UK (CRUK cancerresearchuk.org) found just 48% of those who'd experienced a red flag symptom, such as unexplained weight loss and a new or unusual lump, contacted their GP within half a year.

'You might think of red flag symptoms like coughing up blood or unexplained bleeding as hard to ignore, but this research shows that many do,' says Dr Julie Sharp, CRUK's head of health and patient involvement.

She points out that people from deprived backgrounds in particular face more barriers to seeking help, and stresses: 'Whether it's a red flag symptom or not, if you notice a change to your health that's unusual for you or isn't going away, contact your GP as soon as you can. Your doctor is there for you and wants to hear about any concerns.'

Not telling a doctor about unusual health changes may reduce the chances of an early cancer diagnosis. When diagnosed at stage one – the earliest stage – more than nine in 10 (92%) people will survive bowel cancer for five years or more. It's one in 10 (10%) when diagnosed at stage four – the latest stage.

Sharp says anyone who has any of the following symptoms should have them checked by a doctor immediately. She stresses that in most cases it won't be cancer, but if it is, spotting it early can make a real difference and possibly save your life.

1. Unexplained pain

Pain is a sign that something's wrong, and while it's easy to just hope it'll go away, if it persists it's important to get it checked out. 'As we get older, it's more common to experience aches and pains,' says Sharp. 'But unexplained pain could be a sign of something more serious.'

2. Heavy night sweats

Sharp says there are many reasons you might sweat at night, including infections, certain medications, or going through the menopause. However, very heavy, drenching night sweats can also be a sign of several cancers, including leukaemia and lymphoma.

3. Unexplained weight loss

There are, of course, many reasons for unexplained weight loss other than cancer, including gut and thyroid problems. But Sharp says that while small weight changes over time are normal, if you lose a noticeable amount of weight without trying to, you should tell your doctor.

4. Unusual lumps or swelling

Lumps are one of the most well-known cancer symptoms, and while they can be caused by many less serious issues like an injury, Sharp stresses that persistent lumps or swelling in any part of the body, including the neck, armpit, stomach, groin, chest, breast or testicle, should be taken seriously.

5. Fatigue

Tiredness can, of course, be caused by many things, including stress, auto-immune problems, or simply having trouble sleeping. 'But if you're feeling tired for no clear reason, it could be a sign that something is wrong,' says Sharp.

6. Unexplained bleeding

Unexplained bleeding in poo, wee or vomit, coughing up blood, or any unexplained vaginal bleeding between periods, after sex or after the menopause, should be checked by a doctor, says Sharp, who explains that the blood may look red, brown or black. Such bleeding can often be caused by something far less serious than cancer, but you should always report it to your doctor, she stresses.

7. Skin changes

These can include a sore that won't heal, a new mole or changes to a mole's size, shape or colour, plus crustiness, itching or bleeding. Look at what doctors call the ABCDE Checklist to help you spot key changes. In addition, Sharp says any unusual change in a patch of skin or a nail should be checked by a doctor.

8. Digestive and eating problems

Problems including difficulty swallowing, unusual heartburn or indigestion or appetite loss can be red flag symptoms of cancer, says Sharp, although they can also be caused by lots of other things, including gastro-oesophageal reflux disease (GORD), stomach ulcers, or simply eating a spicy meal. But swallowing problems that don't go away may be a sign of head and neck cancers, and persistent indigestion that can't be explained could be a sign of a number of cancers including pancreatic, stomach and oesophageal.

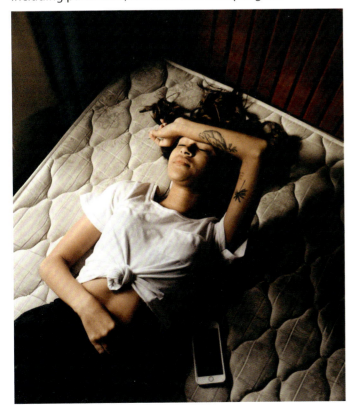

Appetite loss is also a sign of many different cancers, and Sharp says 'Appetite loss can happen for many different reasons – speak to your doctor if you've noticed you're not as hungry as usual and it's not getting any better.'

9. Hoarse voice, cough or breathlessness

It's really common to have a hoarse voice if you've had a cold, but the NHS says if you're hoarse for more than three weeks you should see a doctor, as it's a possible sign of throat cancer. Similarly, Sharp says if you have an unexplained cough that doesn't go away in a few weeks or gets worse, it could be a sign of lung cancer, and if you're getting more breathless than usual, tell your doctor – while it might just be related to an infection or other heart or lung problems, it could be a cancer sign.

10. Toileting changes

Sharp says if you experience a change in bowel habits including constipation, looser poo or pooing more often, having problems weeing, such as needing to go more often or urgently, experiencing pain when weeing, or not being able to go when you need to, or if there's blood in your wee or poo, you should see a doctor. While such symptoms could be a sign of bowel or bladder cancer, they could easily be something far less serious. Sharp says: 'These symptoms can all be caused by conditions other than cancer, but it's best to get them checked out.'

11. Persistent mouth ulcer

Although mouth ulcers are common, especially when you're run down, they usually get better within about two weeks. But Sharp says an ulcer or red or white patch that doesn't heal after three weeks should be reported to your doctor or dentist.

12. Unusual breast changes

It's not just a lump that can be a breast cancer symptom – look out for any change in the size, shape or feel of your breast, or any skin changes, redness, or pain in the breast. Sharp says fluid – which may be blood-stained – leaking from the nipple could also be a sign of cancer.

13. Persistent bloating

Bloating is another symptom that's very common and usually not serious. However, while Sharp says it's common to experience a bloated or swollen tummy that comes and goes, if you feel bloated most days, even if it's intermittent, talk to your doctor. Bloating can be a sign of several cancers, but particularly ovarian.

26 April 2023

How do I check for cancer?

- It's good to be aware of what your body usually looks and feels like. But there's no need to check yourself at a set time or in a set way.

- If you notice anything unusual for you, listen to your body and tell your doctor.

- Spotting cancer at an early stage can save lives.

This article has advice on self-checking for cancer. Our advice is based on the best scientific studies that look at lots of people over long periods of time. Some of it may surprise you or be different to what you were told in the past. But the best research shows that there's no one way to check your body for cancer. And people who self-check regularly are no more likely to survive cancer. So there is no need to check yourself regularly at a set time or in a set way.

We talk about breasts or chest, and testicles in more detail on this page because people often ask if they should check these body parts.

Should I check my body for cancer?

Lots of people talk about doing 'self-checks' (also known as self-examinations or self-exams) at home, to try and spot cancer early. But there's no good evidence to suggest that regularly self-checking any part of your body at a set time or set way is helpful. It can actually do more harm than good, by picking up things that wouldn't have gone on to cause you problems. This can lead to unnecessary tests or treatment, that may have side effects and cause worry.

If you know what's normal for you, it's easier to notice if anything changes. So instead of regular self-checks, be aware of what is normal for you and listen to your body if it's telling you something isn't right.

'The advice now is not to be fixated on checking on a regular basis – unless you've been told to do so by a healthcare professional,' says Dr Ameesh Patel, North East London GP and Havering North Primary Care Network Cancer Lead.

'You should be body aware, which means you should be aware, from a young age, of your body appearance and what the feel of your body is, and then you have a good baseline of normality for you'

Self-checking is different to cancer screening. Screening is a test that looks for early signs of cancer in people without symptoms.

What should I look for?

There are over 200 signs and symptoms of cancer so it's not possible to remember them all. It's also not your job to know what's wrong. Some common cancer symptoms are easy to see, but others can happen inside your body making them difficult to see or touch. So, the best thing you can do is to tell your doctor if you notice anything that's not normal for you. In most cases it won't be cancer – but if it is, spotting it early can make a real difference.

Should I check my breasts or chest?

It is good to be breast aware. This means knowing what your breasts or chest usually look and feel like, so you know what's normal for you. This includes knowing what your breasts are like at different times of the month. But you do not need to check your breasts or chest at a set time or in a set way.

Research has shown that women who regularly self-check their breasts aren't any less likely to die from breast cancer. But they are almost twice as likely to have an unnecessary test (biopsy) on a lump that turns out not to be cancer.

Remember, it's still important to listen to your body and tell your doctor if you've noticed any unusual lumps or other changes to your chest, breasts or nipples that aren't normal for you. If something's not quite right (no matter how you find it), get it checked out.

Should I check my testicles?

It's a good idea to know what your testicles usually look and feel like, and to be aware of their normal size and weight. This can make it easier to spot unusual changes, which you should always tell your doctor about.

But there's no need to regularly self-check at a set time or in a set way, as there is a lack of evidence showing a benefit to testicular self-checking.

Remember, it's still important to listen to your body and tell your doctor if you've noticed any unusual lumps, swellings or other changes to your testicles that aren't normal for you. If something's not quite right (no matter how you find it), get it checked out.

17 October 2022

Have you noticed any changes in your health?

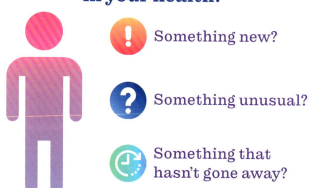

Something new?

Something unusual?

Something that hasn't gone away?

Spotting cancer at an early stage means treatment is more likely to be successful.

If you notice anything that's not normal for you, contact your GP practice.

Source: Cancer Research UK

How should I check my breasts?

There's no right or wrong way to check your breasts. But it's important to know how your breasts usually look and feel. That way, you can spot any changes quickly and report them to a GP.

Be breast aware

Every woman's breasts are different in terms of size, shape and consistency. It's also possible for one breast to be larger than the other.

Get used to how your breasts feel at different times of the month. This can change during your menstrual cycle. For example, some women have tender and lumpy breasts, especially near the armpit, around the time of their period.

After the menopause, normal breasts feel softer, less firm and not as lumpy.

The NHS Breast Screening Programme has produced a 5-point plan for being breast aware:

1. know what's normal for you
2. look at your breasts and feel them
3. know what changes to look for
4. report any changes to a GP without delay
5. attend routine screening if you're aged 50 to 70

Look at your breasts and feel each breast and armpit, and up to your collarbone. You may find it easiest to do this in the shower or bath, by running a soapy hand over each breast and up under each armpit.

You can also look at your breasts in the mirror. Look with your arms by your side and also with them raised.

Breast changes to look out for

See a GP if you notice any of the following changes:

- a change in the size, outline or shape of your breast
- a change in the look or feel of the skin on your breast, such as puckering or dimpling, a rash or redness
- a new lump, swelling, thickening or bumpy area in one breast or armpit that was not there before
- a discharge of fluid from either of your nipples
- any change in nipple position, such as your nipple being pulled in or pointing differently
- a rash (like eczema), crusting, scaly or itchy skin or redness on or around your nipple
- any discomfort or pain in one breast, particularly if it's a new pain and does not go away (although pain is only a symptom of breast cancer in rare cases)

Always see a GP if you are concerned

Breast changes can happen for many reasons, and most of them are not serious. Lots of women have breast lumps, and most breast lumps are not cancerous.

However, if you find changes in your breast that are not normal for you, it's best to see a GP as soon as possible. This is because it's important to rule out breast cancer. If cancer is detected, then appropriate treatment should be planned as quickly as possible.

22 July 2021

Changes to look for

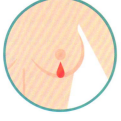
Nipple discharge

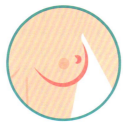
Lumping or thickening

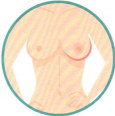
Skin texture change

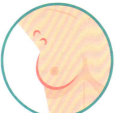
Armpit pain

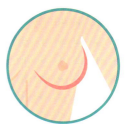
Change in how the nipple looks

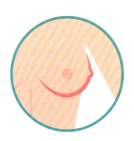
Visible lump

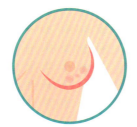
Dimpling

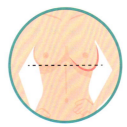
Pulled in nipple

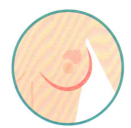
Skin irritation

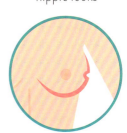
Skin dimpling

How to check your balls

It's time to build a better relationship with your body – starting with the testicles.

Check your balls, you guys. Check. Your. Balls.

Or, C.Y.B. – It's not a thing, YET, but we're going to make it one.

While you may be being encouraged to stop playing with your private parts in some contexts, we are encouraging you to do the exact opposite here. And it's for your own good.

But why?

When was the last time you checked your balls to see how they're doing?

If it was recently – keep doing it; if you've not done it before – it's not too late to start.

It's all about building a relationship with your balls. It sounds ridiculous to say it, but it's a very easy (and necessary) thing to do. You already see them every day. You already touch them every day. You already clean them every day* (*we sincerely hope).

So, why not use one of the opportunities to give them a good check to see if they're healthy?

We're asking you this because testicular cancer is the most common cancer of men aged between 25 and 49. But it happens to younger and older guys too. So, a simple ball-check will give you the best chance of beating the disease should it ever happen to you.

We're not saying you need to do it every day; more like once a month. It's the best way to notice if there are any changes over time to your testicles – changes which would indicate a lot about your health.

Like a new lump, bump, or swelling. It's about noticing a change, something different than before. Simple as that. So check your balls.

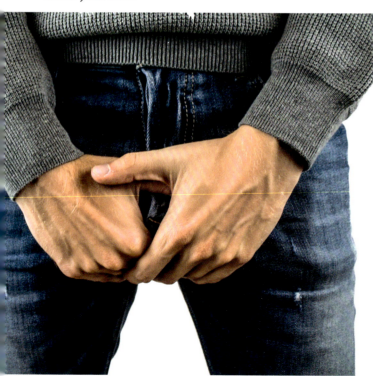

Ok, so what's the story?

Although most cancers get more common as you get older, testicular cancer is different. It's most likely to happen when you're young or middle aged.

Cancer can be a scary word, but the stats are favourable on this one. According to the Teenage Cancer Trust, the chances of making a full recovery from testicular cancer are good, but finding it early makes it a lot easier to treat.

In short, more than 98% of men who get testicular cancer will be cured.

How do I go about this then?

You don't need to 'grow a pair', but instead just 'grab a pair*' (*your own pair, of course.)

It's a good practice to get into, so just work it into your routine. Doing it after a bath or shower is best, because the skin around your balls is loose and relaxed.

Rest your balls in the palm of your hand, and gently roll each one between finger and thumb. What you're looking for may include: 1) a lump (which might be painless); 2) increased size; 3) hardness; or 4) pain or heaviness in the ball sack.

And just so you know, it's normal to have one ball slightly bigger, or hanging slightly lower than the other. That's why you should get to know what's normal for you and then look for changes over time.

If you find something strange, don't stew over it, or worry about it. Just get an appointment with your doctor as soon as you can – they're there to help, not to scare you.

Remember: ball problems are usually caused by something much less serious than cancer, so it's best to put your mind to rest. And doctors are the best placed people to figure out what's wrong, so don't try and figure it out yourself.

Any more information?

It's all about taking pride in yourself and getting to know your body. I mean, if not already (which is totally fine), you're probably already interested, or becoming interested in what's between other people's legs, so why not familiarise yourself with what's between yours along the way? It's a good habit to get into.

Here's some of the best resources for further reading on how to check your balls:

- NHS
- It's In The Bag
- Teenage Cancer Trust

Oh and CYB.

Yup, still trying to make it a thing!

The above information is reprinted with kind permission from Fumble.
© 2023 Fumble

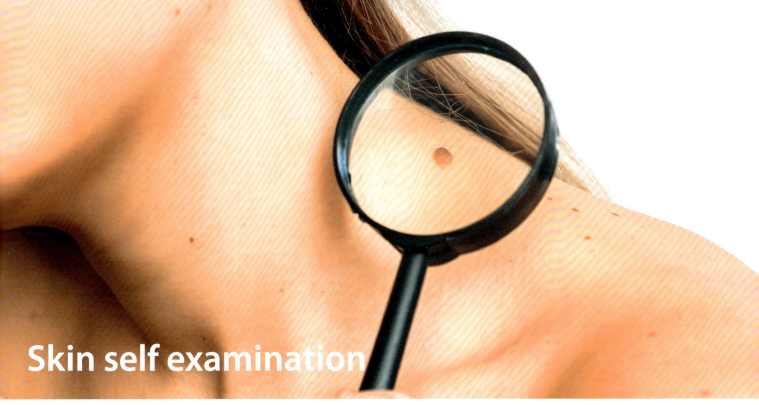

Skin self examination

We recommend that you do a head-to-toe self-examination of your skin every month. This way you can find any new or changing lesions that might be cancerous or precancerous.

Performed regularly, self-examination can alert you to changes in your skin and aid in the early detection of skin cancer. It should be done often enough to become a habit, but not so often as to feel like a bother. For most people, once a month is ideal, but ask your doctor if you should do more frequent checks.

You may find it helpful to have a doctor do a full-body exam first, to assure you that any existing spots, freckles, or moles are normal or treat any that may not be.

After the first few times, self-examination should take no more than 10 minutes — a small investment in what could be a life-saving procedure.

There are three main types of skin cancer: basal cell carcinoma, squamous cell carcinoma, and melanoma. Because each has many different appearances, it is important to know the early warning signs. Look especially for a change of any kind.

Do not ignore a suspicious spot simply because it does not hurt. Skin cancers may be painless, but dangerous all the same. If you notice one or more of the warning signs, see a doctor right away, preferably one who specializes in diseases of the skin.

- A skin growth that increases in size and appears pearly, translucent, tan, brown, black, or multicolored

- A mole, birthmark, beauty mark, or any brown spot that:

  - changes color

  - increases in size or thickness

  - changes in texture

  - is irregular in outline

  - is bigger than 6mm or 1/4"; the size of a pencil eraser

  - appears after age 21

- A spot or sore that continues to itch, hurt, crust, scab, erode or bleed

- An open sore that does not heal within three weeks

Don't overlook it. Don't delay. See a physician, preferably one who specializes in diseases of the skin, if you note any change in an existing mole, freckle, or spot or if you find a new one with any of the warning signs of skin cancer.

About 90 percent of non-melanoma skin cancers are associated with exposure to ultraviolet (UV) radiation from the sun. We always recommended using a sunscreen with an SPF 30 or higher as one important part of a complete sun protection regimen. Sunscreen alone is not enough.

Skin cancer prevention tips:

- Seek the shade, especially between 10 AM and 4 PM. Do not burn.

- Avoid tanning and UV tanning booths.

- Cover up with clothing, including a broad-brimmed hat and UV-blocking sunglasses.

- Use a broad-spectrum (UVA/UVB) sunscreen with an SPF of 30 or higher every day.

- For extended outdoor activity, use a water-resistant, broad-spectrum (UVA/UVB) sunscreen with an SPF of 30 or higher.

- Apply 1 ounce (2 tablespoons) of sunscreen to your entire body 30 minutes before going outside. Reapply every two hours or immediately after swimming or excessive sweating.

- Keep newborns out of the sun. Sunscreens should be used on babies over the age of six months.

- Examine your skin head-to-toe every month.

- See your physician every year for a professional skin exam.

The 'ABCDE' rule

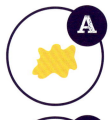

Asymmetry
An asymmetrical mole should be shown to your doctor

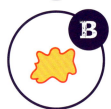

Border
A mole with uneven border should be shown to your doctor

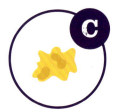

Colour
Moles with two or more colours should be shown to your doctor

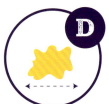

Diameter
Moles larger than 5mm should be shown to your doctor

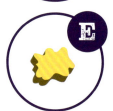

Elevation
A mole that is becoming raised should be shown to your doctor

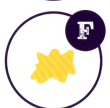

Firm
A mole that feels firm or solid should be shown to your doctor

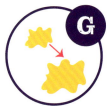

Growing
A mole that is showing signs of change should be shown to your doctor

Source: Melanoma UK

The ABCDE Rule of skin cancer is an easy-to-remember system for determining whether a mole or growth may be cancerous.

When a doctor performs a skin check, they look at every lump, spot and mole on your entire body; areas of concern are assessed for signs of skin cancer using the ABCDE method of melanoma detection.

As kids we are taught to 'slip, slop, slap, seek and slide' but not that much about the ABCs of skin cancer - a simple process that allows anyone to check their skin for the warning signs of skin cancer.

If you see two or more warning signs, consult a doctor without delay. It may be nothing, but it's always better to be safe than sorry. Skin cancer, both melanoma and non-melanoma, can usually be treated successfully if caught early.

The above information is reprinted with kind permission from Melanoma UK.
© 2023 Melanoma UK

www.melanomauk.org.uk

Prevention is the best medicine – what to expect from your smear test

Cervical cancer screenings save at least 2,000 lives every year in the UK. Here's what you should expect from your smear test and why these screenings are important.

One in 142 women in the UK will be diagnosed with cervical cancer in their lifetime. A cervical cancer screening, better known as a smear test, can detect the development of abnormal cells in the cervix and prevent cervical cancer.

Who is eligible?

All women and people with a cervix are eligible for a cervical cancer screening. This includes Trans men and non-binary people who are assigned female at birth and registered with their GP as female.

Screenings will occur at regular intervals between the ages of 25 and 64. If you're 25 to 49, invites to screenings will be every three years. For those aged 50 to 64, this will be every five years.

What to expect

A smear test should take around five minutes, and the whole appointment should take at most ten minutes. A female GP or nurse will carry out the test, but if you have any concerns, contact your GP practice or sexual health clinic ahead of your appointment, and they will work with you.

The smear test may feel uncomfortable, but it should not be painful. If you experience pain during the exam, inform the GP or nurse attending you immediately.

Many people put off booking or attending their smear test because they're not sure what to expect. Healthcare professionals conducting the exam will ensure you feel comfortable and safe and will be happy to talk you through the procedure.

Talk to someone

A smear test is a very personal procedure, which can be off-putting for some. You can talk to someone about the test if you feel embarrassed or worried. Sometimes it's easier to speak to someone you don't know. Your GP or nurse can talk you through what to expect, addressing any concerns or worries about the test.

You may want to contact an organisation that provides information and support about having cervical screening if you're unable to speak with your practice:

Eve Appeal offers information and support for anyone affected by gynaecological cancers. It also provides information about cervical screening for transgender, non-binary and intersex people. Call their helpline on 0808 802 0019.

Jo's Cervical Cancer Trust (Jo's Trust) offers information and support for anyone affected by cervical cancer or abnormal cervical cell changes. Call their helpline on 0808 802 8000.

After the exam

Your GP practice or sexual health clinic will send your cell sample to a lab after the test. Ask the nurse or doctor when you will get your test results. Often, the most challenging part of cervical screening is waiting for results. It is natural to worry about this.

Usually, you will get a letter with the results within two to four weeks. If you are still waiting to hear something by six weeks, tell your GP so they can check for you.

After the exam, you may experience light vaginal bleeding for a day. If it continues longer than this or is particularly heavy, contact your GP or sexual health clinic immediately.

Where can I get a smear test?

Your GP practice can offer you an appointment for your smear test. You will be automatically invited to a test up to six months before you turn 25 or when your next one is due.

However, the impact of the pandemic may mean that you are overdue an appointment or have yet to receive an invite. It's always worthwhile checking in with your GP.

You can also attend a sexual health clinic to have your smear test done if your GP practice cannot offer you an appointment.

20 January 2023

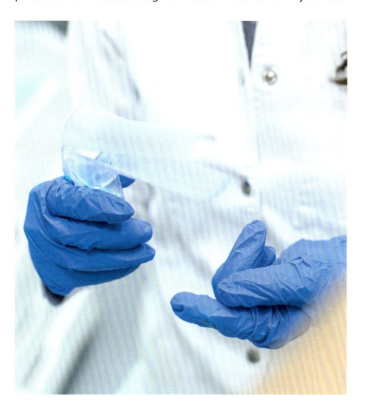

HPV vaccine reduces cervical cancer by 87%

The human papillomavirus (HPV) vaccine reduces cervical cancer rates by 87% in women who were offered the jab between the ages of 12-13, confirms a new study.

Researchers from King's found the HPV vaccination programme prevented around 450 cervical cancers and around 17,200 pre-cancers by the middle of 2019. They also found cervical cancer rates were reduced by 62% in women offered vaccination between the ages of 14-16, and 34% in women aged 16-18 when they were offered the jab.

The paper, published today in the *Lancet* and funded by Cancer Research UK, looked at all cervical cancers diagnosed in England in women aged 20-64 between January 2006 and June 2019. Three of these cohorts formed the vaccinated population, where women were vaccinated with Cervarix between the ages of 12-13, 14-16 and 16-18 respectively. Incidences of cervical cancer and non-invasive cervical carcinoma (CIN3) in the seven populations were recorded separately.

The vaccine programme started in England in 2008 and at the time used the bivalent vaccine, Cervarix, which protects against the two most common types of HPV. Since September 2012 the quadrivalent vaccine Gardasil has been used instead.

Almost all cervical cancers are caused by HPV. The vaccine is most effective when given before sexual activity when people are unlikely to have been exposed to HPV. The virus is linked to other cancers including vaginal, vulval, anal, penile and some head and neck cancers.

He added: 'Assuming most people continue to get the HPV vaccine and go for screening, cervical cancer will become a rare disease. This year we have already seen the power of vaccines in controlling the COVID-19 pandemic. These data show that vaccination works in preventing some cancers.'

Dr Vanessa Saliba, Consultant Epidemiologist in Immunisations at Public Health England, said: 'These remarkable findings confirm that the HPV vaccine saves lives by dramatically reducing cervical cancer rates among women. This reminds us that vaccines are one of the most important tools we have to help us live longer, healthier lives.

'This fantastic achievement has been made possible thanks to the high uptake of the HPV vaccine in England. We encourage all who are eligible for the HPV vaccine to take it up when it is offered in school. All those eligible can catch-up until their 25th birthday. Together with cervical screening, this will help to protect more women from preventable cases of cervical cancer.

4 November 2021

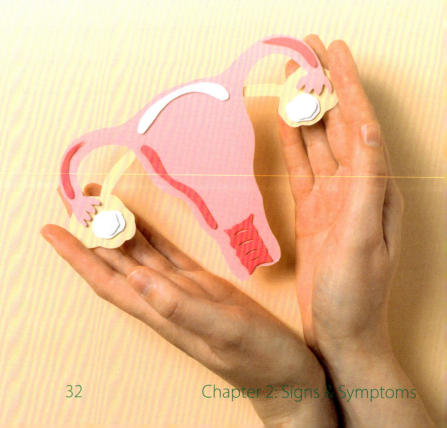

'It's been incredible to see the impact of HPV vaccination, and now we can prove it prevented hundreds of women from developing cancer in England. We've known for many years that HPV vaccination is very effective in preventing particular strains of the virus, but to see the real-life impact of the vaccine has been truly rewarding.'

– Professor Peter Sasieni, lead author from the School of Cancer and Pharmaceutical Sciences

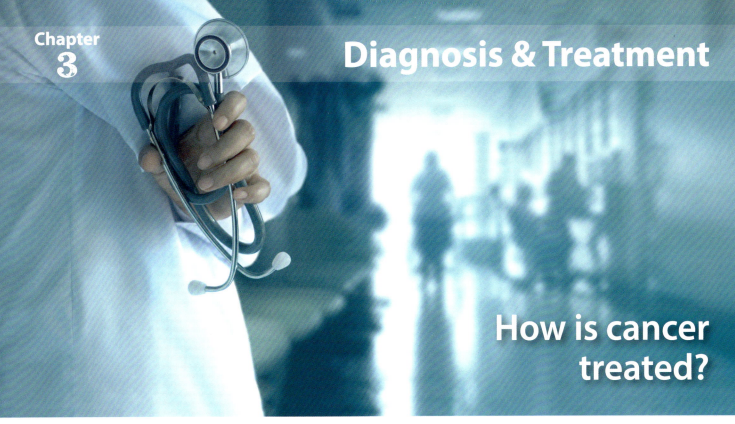

How is cancer treated?

There are several types of cancer treatment. It's common for a combination of treatments to be used. You may be offered treatment as part of a clinical trial.

Treatments include:

- surgery – an operation to remove the cancer is the main treatment for many types of cancer

- radiotherapy – high energy X-rays are used to destroy the cancer cells

- chemotherapy – uses anti-cancer (cytotoxic) drugs to destroy cancer cells

- hormonal therapy – reduces the level of hormones in the body or blocks hormones from reaching cancer cells

- targeted therapies – destroy cancer cells, usually by interfering with the cancer's ability to grow

- stem cell or bone marrow treatments – allow high doses of anti-cancer treatment to be given or are used to give the person a new immune system to fight the cancer

You may also be given supportive treatments to treat side effects. Supportive treatments include:

- treatments to treat or reduce the risk of infection

- steroids

- blood transfusions

- bone strengthening treatments

Some people use complementary therapies, such as massage or relaxation therapies, as well as conventional medical treatments. Complementary therapies do not claim to treat cancer. But, some people may use them to boost their physical or emotional health or to relieve symptoms or side effects. Always tell your doctor if you are thinking about using complementary therapies. Although many are safe to use alongside conventional treatment, some may not be suitable.

Clinical trials research new treatments to see if they are more effective than the standard treatments already available. This may be testing a new drug, researching different ways of carrying out an operation or a new way of giving treatment. They aim to find the treatments that work best and cause the fewest side effects.

Surgery

Surgery is one of the main treatments for cancer and can be used for lots of reasons. Surgery can be used to:

- diagnose cancer

- remove cancer

- find out how big the cancer is and if it has spread to other parts of the body

- control symptoms of cancer

- restore parts of the body (for example breast reconstruction)

Surgery can cure many cancers.

The type of surgery you have will depend on the cancer that is treated. Your doctor or nurse can give you specific information about your surgery.

Radiotherapy

Radiotherapy uses high-energy rays to treat disease. It can be given both externally and internally.

External radiotherapy aims high-energy X-rays at the affected area using a large machine.

Internal radiotherapy involves having radioactive material placed inside the body. You can be given radiotherapy for different reasons. Doctors can give radiotherapy to try and destroy a tumour and cure the cancer. This is called curative treatment. It may be used with other treatments, such as surgery or chemotherapy.

If it's not possible to cure the cancer, doctors may give you radiotherapy to help relieve symptoms you have. This is called palliative treatment.

Radiotherapy works by destroying cancer cells in the area that's being treated. Normal cells can also be damaged by radiotherapy, which may cause side effects. Cancer cells cannot repair themselves after radiotherapy, but normal cells usually can.

The type of radiotherapy you're given will depend on the type of cancer you have and your individual situation.

Chemotherapy

Chemotherapy uses anti-cancer (cytotoxic) drugs to destroy cancer cells. The drugs also affect healthy cells, causing side effects such as feeling sick or an increased risk of infection.

Unlike cancer cells these cells usually repair themselves. Most side effects improve when treatment is finished.

Chemotherapy can be given as a main treatment or after other treatments to reduce the risk of the cancer coming back. Or, you may have it to shrink a cancer before surgery or radiotherapy. It is sometimes used at the same time as radiotherapy (chemoradiation).

Chemotherapy is also given to control cancer that has spread and to relieve symptoms.

The chemotherapy you have will depend on different things, such as the cancer type, the risk of it coming back, or whether it has spread. Some people have tests during treatment to check if the cancer is responding to chemotherapy.

You usually have chemotherapy by injection or a 'drip' into a vein, or as tablets. Sometimes, it's given in other ways, such as into the spine or into the bladder, depending on the type of cancer.

Targeted therapies

Targeted therapies (sometimes known as biological therapies) can be used to stimulate the immune system, control the growth of cancer cells or to overcome side effects of treatment.

There are several types of targeted treatment:

- monoclonal antibodies
- cancer growth inhibitors
- angiogenesis inhibitors
- vaccines

Hormonal therapy

Hormones are substances produced naturally in the body. They act as chemical messengers and influence the growth and activity of cells. Hormones are produced by a number of different organs and glands, which together are known as the endocrine system.

Hormonal therapies work by altering the production or activity of particular hormones in the body. They are most commonly used to treat breast cancer and prostate cancer. The type of hormone therapy given depends on the type of cancer being treated.

There are several different types of hormonal therapy. They are usually given as either tablets or injections. The side effects will vary and depend on the individual drug. General side effects can include tiredness, headaches, feeling sick and muscle or joint aches.

Stem cells

Stem cells are blood cells at their earliest stage of development. All blood cells develop from stem cells. Bone marrow is a spongy material inside the bones. The bone marrow is where stem cells are made.

There are 2 different types of stem cell transplants:

- high-dose treatment with stem cell support
- allogenic (donor) stem cell transplants

A transplant using stem cells (early blood cells) from another person (a donor) is called a donor stem cell transplant. The medical term for this is an allogeneic transplant. It's also sometimes called an allograft or a bone marrow transplant.

A donor stem cell transplant can be used to treat cancers such as lymphoma, myeloma and leukaemia. It's also sometimes used to treat some other diseases of the bone marrow or immune system.

The aim of a donor stem cell transplant is to replace your bone marrow and immune system with that of a donor's. This will give you a new, healthy bone marrow, and an immune system that can fight any remaining cancer cells.

High-dose treatments

High-dose treatment with stem cell support is normally given after treatment with standard chemotherapy. It's used to destroy any remaining cancer cells and can increase the chances of curing certain types of cancers or leukaemias.

High-dose treatment with stem cell support involves storing your stem cells and returning them to you after treatment. This allows you to have much higher doses of chemotherapy than usual.

This treatment is also called autologous stem cell transplant. It is used to treat different cancers and some types of leukaemias and lymphomas. It can also be used to treat some rare non-cancerous conditions.

3 November 2022

www.nhsinform.scot

Cancer waiting times

There are waiting time targets for the diagnosis and treatment of cancer in the different UK nations.

Having to wait

Getting a diagnosis of cancer can sometimes take a while. Sometimes it might feel that you are waiting too long. Usually, everyone will have to wait for appointments and to have tests or get results. Only then you can start treatment. This can be frustrating and difficult to cope with.

You may begin to worry that the cancer will spread during this time. But we know that most cancers usually grow slowly. So waiting a few weeks for a scan or treatment does not usually affect how well the treatment works.

The different UK nations have their targets around:

* referral for suspected cancer

* waiting times to a diagnosis

* waiting times to start treatment

Urgent referral for suspected cancer

Your GP, dentist or nurse will arrange your referral to see a hospital doctor (specialist), or to have tests. They should tell you if this is an urgent referral for suspected cancer. An urgent referral can be worrying. But remember that more than 9 in every 10 people (more than 90%) referred this way will not have a diagnosis of cancer.

In England, an urgent referral means that you should see a specialist within 2 weeks. In Northern Ireland, the 2 week wait only applies for suspected breast cancer.

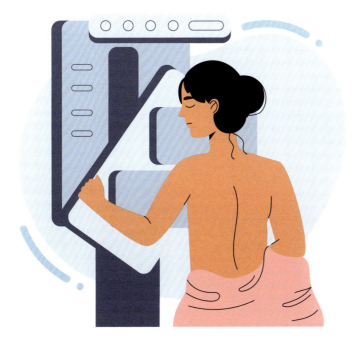

Scotland, Wales and (in general) Northern Ireland don't have the 2 week time frame to see a specialist. But wherever you live, a specialist will see you as soon as possible.

Waiting for tests

A specialist may need to do a variety of tests to decide on a diagnosis. If they diagnose cancer, you may then need further tests. This is to get as much information about the cancer as possible.

For example, your specialist might arrange a scan such as a CT scan, MRI scan or PET scan. This helps them to work out the stage of the cancer. The stage of the cancer refers to the size and whether it has spread. This helps your medical team to decide which treatment is best for you.

Unfortunately, you might have to wait for an appointment for some of these tests. This could be because of the high number of people needing certain scans.

Some types of specialised scans are only available in larger hospitals. So you might need to go to another hospital for your scan, which can increase the length of time you wait.

Waiting for scan results

A specialist doctor needs to examine your scan and write a report. They send the report to your cancer specialist who will give you the results. It usually takes a couple of weeks for the results to come through. But it might be ready sooner if your specialist puts urgent on the scan request form.

Waiting for results can make you anxious. Ask your specialist to give you a rough idea of how long your test results are likely to take. You can ring their secretary if you have not heard anything after a couple of weeks.

Waiting for a diagnosis

England

NHS England has introduced a new target called the Faster Diagnosis Standard (FDS). The target is that you should not wait more than 28 days from referral to finding out whether you have cancer or not. This is to make sure patients don't have to wait too long to find out their diagnosis.

The FDS applies to those people who are referred:

* by their GP for suspected cancer

* by their GP with breast symptoms where cancer is not suspected

* following an abnormal screening result from a cancer screening test

The 3 screening programmes in England are:

- breast cancer
- bowel cancer
- cervical screening

Scotland, Northern Ireland and Wales

Scotland, Northern Ireland and Wales do not have a Faster Diagnosis Standard target.

Waiting to start treatment

There are waiting time targets to start treatment.

In England, Scotland and Northern Ireland the current targets are:

- no more than 2 months (62 days) wait between the date the hospital receives an urgent referral for suspected cancer and the start of treatment
- no more than 31 days wait between the meeting at which you and your doctor agree the treatment plan and the start of treatment

In May 2019 Wales introduced the Single Cancer Pathway. This combines all urgent and non urgent referrals into one target time of 62 days or less. This means, that when cancer is first suspected, everyone should have a confirmed diagnosis and start treatment within 62 days.

The time starts from one of the following:

- when you first see your GP and they suspect cancer
- when you have a suspicious change on your screening mammogram and you need further tests

If your cancer comes back

NHS England has a waiting time target for cancer that has come back (a recurrence). They say that you should start treatment within 31 days. This time starts from the meeting in which you and your doctor have agreed your treatment plan.

Scotland, Wales and Northern Ireland have not set this target. But you will start treatment as soon as possible.

A new primary cancer

In some situations, your doctor may diagnose a new primary cancer instead of a recurrence. If so, you should wait no more than 2 months (62 days) to start treatment. This time starts on the date that the hospital has received an urgent referral for suspected cancer.

You might have to wait longer if you need extra tests to diagnose your cancer. Waiting times can vary depending on the type of cancer and the type of treatment you are going to have.

Tell your specialist or nurse if you worry about waiting for treatment. They will understand that you find it hard to wait a few weeks for treatment. They will be able to reassure you. Usually, waiting should not affect how well your treatment works.

20 July 2022

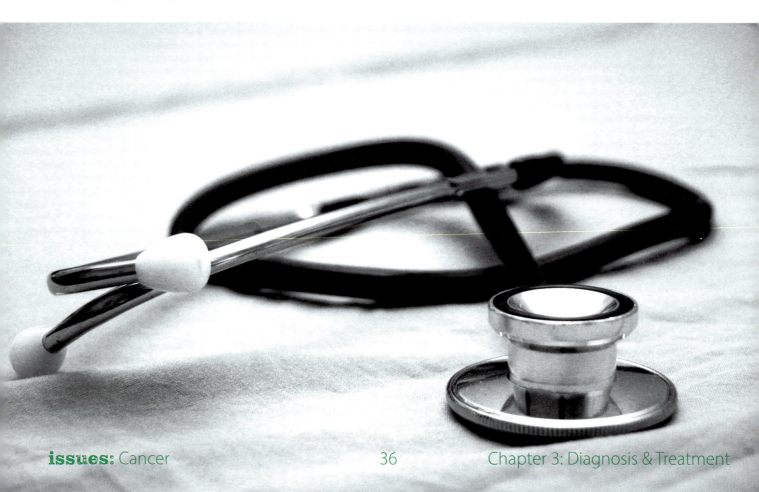

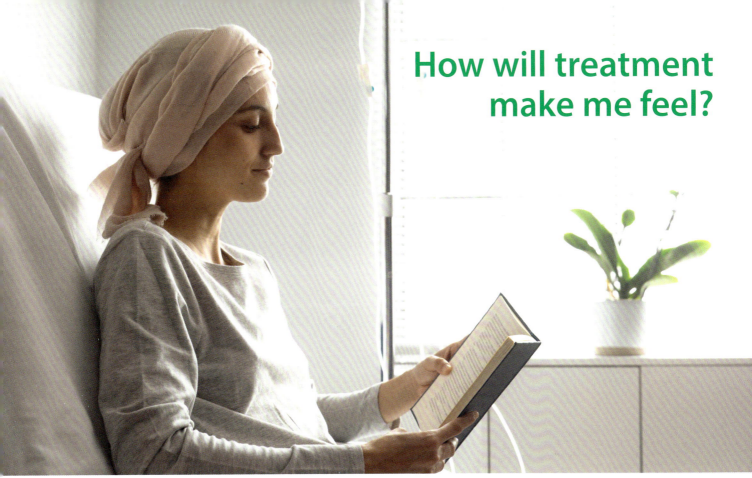

How will treatment make me feel?

Cancer treatment can be tough. But not all people react the same way to treatment. Some side-effects are worse than others and you may experience some or all of them. If you are suffering, tell your doctor as there are usually lots of things they can do to make it easier on you.

On the plus side, most effects are short-term and will usually get better once treatment ends. Some, are longer lasting and you will find that the team that is caring for you will explain these to you.

So, what things might you experience? Here, we talk about some of the things you may worry about during treatment.

Feeling tired

Tiredness or fatigue is a common side-effect of cancer treatments. But it's not surprising really, as you are mentally, emotionally and physically going through a lot.

If fatigue is affecting you, try to keep track of when it hits. You may find that you are simply trying to do too much and just need to take some time out. Speak to your nurse or doctor if things aren't improving after rest.

Usually, fatigue goes away quite soon after finishing cancer treatment, but it can sometimes take a year to get back to normal.

Chemo brain

Along with fatigue, chemo brain, or brain fog may make you feel that you're struggling to remember things or think clearly. Again, self-care is a good way to help cope with this.

Keep yourself mentally-stimulated by playing puzzles such as crosswords or sudoku. These will also help to pass some of the time you may be spending waiting around in hospital.

Feeling sick

Lots of cancer medication can cause nausea (feeling sick) and sickness. However, there are medicines called anti emetics that will be prescribed to you if your treatment is likely to make you feel, or be sick. Anxiety can also cause nausea, so if you experience this then tell your doctor who will be able to prescribe other suitable medications.

Appetite changes

You may feel that you don't want to eat, or that your favourite food no longer tastes the same. Sometimes, your family may be worried that you are eating, and try to make you eat more, which can just put you off of eating even more!

Make sure that you are still drinking enough liquids, and eat smaller meals and snacks throughout the day rather than three big meals. Eat what you fancy, don't worry about what you should and shouldn't eat. Try to eat higher calorie foods to keep your weight up, or if this isn't possible, you can be given high calorie drinks, which are similar to milkshakes or yogurt.

Changes in taste can also happen. Foods that you usually love may taste strange to you. Try to have strong tasting foods if food is all starting to taste the same. Avoid bland food and add herbs, spices and sauces to make food more interesting.

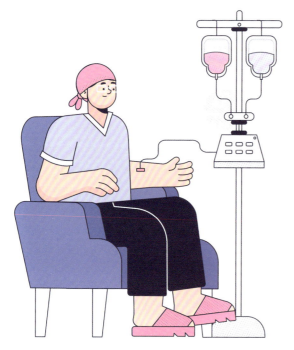

Toilet troubles

Chemotherapy may cause diarrhoea or constipation. Don't be embarrassed about any changes you may have in your toileting habits, there are medications that do help. Don't suffer in silence! Talk to your medical team and they will give you the medication you need.

Sores

Cancer treatment can cause mouth ulcers, a sore mouth and sensitive skin.

Use sensitive skincare products, and build this into your self-care routine so you are keeping your skin in tip-top condition. If you notice anything such as rashes, itchness or anything else that is unusual for you then ask your doctor for advice.

If you have a sore mouth try to keep hydrated as this will help. Also, make sure you are looking after your dental health by brushing regularly and don't skip those dentist appointments.

Your doctor or dentist will be able to advise what to do if you are suffering from mouth ulcers to soothe and help them.

Will I lose my hair?

Some chemotherapy drugs may cause hair loss or thinning. This can be a big worry for lots of people, but there are some things that you can do to help prepare for this. Firstly, check with your doctor to see if hair loss is likely with your treatment. For some types of chemo there are methods to help prevent hair loss by wearing a cold cap, your doctor will be able to advise if this will be suitable for you.

You can also prepare by cutting your hair shorter before treatment as this can stop the weight of the long hair from pulling at the scalp. This may help you to keep your hair a little while longer.

Sometimes, you may feel that you want to wear a wig to hide the hair loss, you may find that you can get help with buying a wig from the NHS or a charity. Alternatively, you could wear hats or scarves or just rock the bald look! Your friends and family may also shave their heads in support or to raise money for charity.

After treatment your hair will start to grow back, it can take about 6 months for a full head of hair, but will be longer until its back to the previous length. Obviously the longer you want your hair the longer it will take! You may find that the new hair growth is a different colour or texture than it was before.

What can I do?

The good news is that there are ways to cope with the side effects of cancer treatment and make them easier to deal with. Some of the things that can help are:

- Talk to your medical care team about your feelings and concerns. They can give you information and advice on how to manage your side effects and what to expect from your treatment.

- Taking medicines or other treatments that can help reduce or prevent some of the side effects. For example, you may take anti-nausea drugs before chemotherapy or use creams or lotions for your skin.

- Eating healthy foods and drinking plenty of fluids to keep your body strong and hydrated.

- Getting enough rest and sleep to help your body heal and recover. You may need to adjust your schedule or activities according to your energy level and mood.

- Doing things that make you happy and relaxed, such as listening to music, reading books, playing games, drawing pictures, or spending time with your family and friends.

- Asking for help and support from your parents, siblings, relatives, teachers, classmates, or other people who care about you. They can help you with your daily tasks, school work, hobbies, or emotions.

- Joining a support group or a counselling program for people with cancer or their family. You can meet other young people who are going through similar situations and share your stories and feelings.

Design

Design a signposting poster with self-care tips for young people with cancer.

What things can they do to help them rest and recuperate?

UEA scientists make breakthrough for 'next generation' cancer treatment

Scientists at the University of East Anglia are a step closer to creating a new generation of light-activated cancer treatments.

The futuristic sounding treatment would work by switching on LED lights embedded close to a tumour, which would then activate biotherapeutic drugs.

These new treatments would be highly targeted and more effective than current state-of-the-art cancer immunotherapies.

New research published today reveals the science behind this innovative idea.

It shows how the UEA team have engineered antibody fragments - which not only 'fuse' with their target but are also light activated.

It means that in future, immunotherapy treatments could be engineered to attack tumours more precisely than ever before.

The principal scientist for this study, Dr Amit Sachdeva, from UEA's School of Chemistry, said: 'Current cancer treatments like chemotherapy kill cancer cells, but they can also damage healthy cells in your body such as blood and skin cells.

'This means that they can cause side effects including hair loss, feeling tired and sick, and they also put patients at increased risk of picking up infections.

'There has therefore been a very big drive to create new treatments that are more targeted and don't have these unwanted side-effects.

'Several antibodies and antibody fragments have already been developed to treat cancer. These antibodies are much more selective than the cytotoxic drugs used in chemotherapy, but they can still cause severe side effects, as antibody targets are also present on healthy cells.'

Now, the UEA team has engineered one of the first antibody fragments that binds to, and forms a covalent bond with, its target - upon irradiation with UV light of a specific wavelength.

Dr Sachdeva said: 'A covalent bond is a bit like melting two pieces of plastic and fusing them together. It means that drug molecules could for example be permanently fixed to a tumour.

'We hope that our work will lead to the development of a new class of highly targeted light-responsive biotherapeutics.

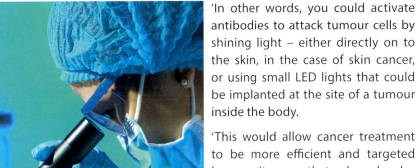

This would mean that antibodies could be activated at the site of a tumour and covalently stick to their target upon light activation.

'In other words, you could activate antibodies to attack tumour cells by shining light – either directly on to the skin, in the case of skin cancer, or using small LED lights that could be implanted at the site of a tumour inside the body.

'This would allow cancer treatment to be more efficient and targeted because it means that only molecules in the vicinity of the tumour would be activated, and it wouldn't affect other cells.

'This would potentially reduce side effects for patients, and also improve antibody residence time in the body.

'It would work for cancers like skin cancer, or where there is a solid tumour – but not for blood cancers like leukaemia.

'Development of these antibody fragments would not have been possible without pioneering work from several other research groups across the globe who developed and optimised methods for site-specific incorporation of non-natural amino acids into proteins expressed in live cells.

'We employed some of these methods to site-specifically install unique light-sensitive amino acids into antibody fragments.'

If the researchers are successful in the next stages of their work, they hope to see the 'next generation' light-activated immunotherapies being used to treat cancer patients within five to 10 years.

This research was funded by the Biotechnology and Biological Sciences Research Council (BBSRC) and the Wellcome Trust. It was led by the University of East Anglia with assistance from the proteomics facility at the John Innes Centre.

'Site-specific encoding of photoactivity and photoreactivity into antibody fragments' is published in the journal *Nature Chemical Biology*.

16 February 2023

Discovery of new T-cell raises prospect of 'universal' cancer therapy

Researchers at Cardiff University have discovered a new type of killer T-cell that offers hope of a 'one-size-fits-all' cancer therapy.

T-cell therapies for cancer - where immune cells are removed, modified and returned to the patient's blood to seek and destroy cancer cells - are the latest paradigm in cancer treatments.

The most widely-used therapy, known as CAR-T, is personalised to each patient but targets only a few types of cancers and has not been successful for solid tumours, which make up the vast majority of cancers.

Cardiff researchers have now discovered T-cells equipped with a new type of T-cell receptor (TCR) which recognises and kills most human cancer types, while ignoring healthy cells.

This TCR recognises a molecule present on the surface of a wide range of cancer cells as well as in many of the body's normal cells but, remarkably, is able to distinguish between healthy cells and cancerous ones, killing only the latter.

The researchers said this meant it offered 'exciting opportunities for pan-cancer, pan-population' immunotherapies not previously thought possible.

How does this new TCR work?

Conventional T-cells scan the surface of other cells to find anomalies and eliminate cancerous cells - which express abnormal proteins - but ignore cells that contain only 'normal' proteins.

The scanning system recognises small parts of cellular proteins that are bound to cell-surface molecules called human leukocyte antigen (HLA), allowing killer T-cells to see what's occurring inside cells by scanning their surface.

HLA varies widely between individuals, which has previously prevented scientists from creating a single T-cell-based treatment that targets most cancers in all people.

But the Cardiff study, published today in Nature Immunology, describes a unique TCR that can recognise many types of cancer via a single HLA-like molecule called MR1.

Unlike HLA, MR1 does not vary in the human population - meaning it is a hugely attractive new target for immunotherapies.

How does the new T-cell work?

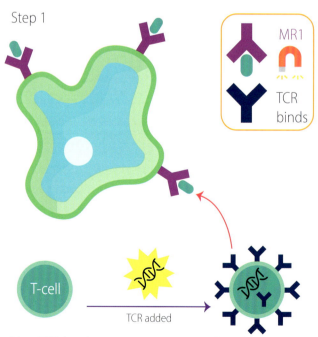

Step 1

MR1
TCR binds

Step 2

TCR binding initiates T-cell attack

T-cell
TCR added
New TCR binds to MR1 on cancer cell surface

Step 3

Cancer cell dies
T-cell is free to patrol and kill other cancer cells

Source: Cardiff University

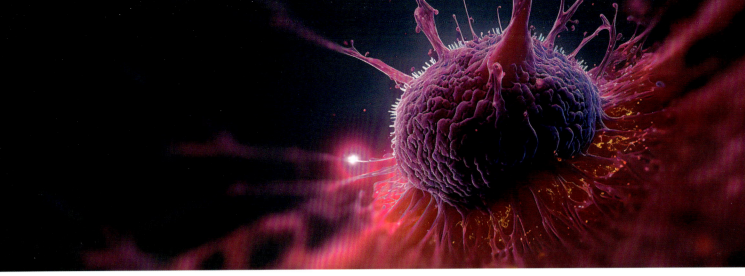

What did the researchers show?

T-cells equipped with the new TCR were shown, in the lab, to kill lung, skin, blood, colon, breast, bone, prostate, ovarian, kidney and cervical cancer cells, while ignoring healthy cells.

To test the therapeutic potential of these cells in vivo, the researchers injected T-cells able to recognise MR1 into mice bearing human cancer and with a human immune system.

This showed 'encouraging' cancer-clearing results which the researchers said was comparable to the now NHS-approved CAR-T therapy in a similar animal model.

The Cardiff group were further able to show that T-cells of melanoma patients modified to express this new TCR could destroy not only the patient's own cancer cells, but also other patients' cancer cells in the laboratory, regardless of the patient's HLA type.

Professor Andrew Sewell, lead author on the study and an expert in T-cells from Cardiff University's School of Medicine, said it was 'highly unusual' to find a TCR with such broad cancer specificity and this raised the prospect of 'universal' cancer therapy.

'We hope this new TCR may provide us with a different route to target and destroy a wide range of cancers in all individuals,' he said.

'Current TCR-based therapies can only be used in a minority of patients with a minority of cancers.'

'Cancer-targeting via MR1-restricted T-cells is an exciting new frontier - it raises the prospect of a 'one-size-fits-all' cancer treatment; a single type of T-cell that could be capable of destroying many different types of cancers across the population.

'Previously nobody believed this could be possible.'

What happens next?

Experiments are under way to determine the precise molecular mechanism by which the new TCR distinguishes between healthy cells and cancer.

The researchers believe it may work by sensing changes in cellular metabolism which causes different metabolic intermediates to be presented at the cancer cell surface by MR1.

The Cardiff group hope to trial this new approach in patients towards the end of this year following further safety testing.

Professor Sewell said a vital aspect of this ongoing safety testing was to further ensure killer T-cells modified with the new TCR recognise cancer cells only.

'There are plenty of hurdles to overcome however if this testing is successful, then I would hope this new treatment could be in use in patients in a few years' time,' he said.

Professor Oliver Ottmann, Cardiff University's Head of Haematology, whose department delivers CAR-T therapy, said: 'This new type of T-cell therapy has enormous potential to overcome current limitations of CAR-T, which has been struggling to identify suitable and safe targets for more than a few cancer types.'

Professor Awen Gallimore, of the University's division of infection and immunity and cancer immunology lead for the Wales Cancer Research Centre, said: 'If this transformative new finding holds up, it will lay the foundation for a "universal" T-cell medicine, mitigating against the tremendous costs associated with the identification, generation and manufacture of personalised T-cells.

'This is truly exciting and potentially a great step forward for the accessibility of cancer immunotherapy.'

The research was funded by the Wellcome Trust, Health and Care Research Wales and Tenovus.

Professor Kieran Walshe, Director of Health and Care Research Wales, said: 'We fund research that aims to make a real difference to people's lives. This study is a significant development in the fight against cancer and it has the potential to transform the treatment of thousands of patients.'

20 January 2020

Further Reading/ Useful Websites

Useful Websites

www.cancerresearchuk.org

www.cardiff.ac.uk

www.fumble.org.uk

www.healthwatch.co.uk

www.imperial.ac.uk

www.independent.co.uk

www.kcl.ac.uk

www.macmillan.org.uk

www.melanomauk.org.uk

www.ndph.ox.ac.uk

www.nhs.uk

www.nhsinform.scot

www.theguardian.com

www.topdoctors.co.uk

www.tyac.org.uk

www.uea.ac.uk

www.ukhsa.blog.gov.uk

www.wcrf-uk.org

Where can I find help?

Below are some telephone numbers, email addresses and websites of agencies or charities that can offer support or advice if you, or someone you know, needs it.

Cancer Research UK
Helpline: 0808 800 4040
www.cancerresearchuk.org

Cancer Help UK
Helpline: 0808 800 4040 to speak to a specialist nurse
www.cancerhelp.org.uk

Children with Cancer UK
Tel: 0800 222 9000
www.childrenwithcancer.org.uk

Jo's Cervical Cancer Trust
Helpline: 0808 802 800
www.jostrust.org.uk

Macmillan Cancer Support
Helpline: 0808 808 0000
www.macmillan.org.uk

Teenagers and Young Adults with Cancer
Tel: 0333 050 7654
Email: info@tyac.org.uk
www.tyac.org.uk

Teenage Cancer Trust
Tel: 020 7612 0370
www.teenagecancertrust.org

Young Lives vs Cancer
Central Support and social care team: 0300 303 5220
Email: GetSupport@younglivesvscancer.org.uk
www.younglivesvscancer.org.uk

There are many different charities that can help support you if you, your family, or your friend has cancer. We have just a few here as an example. There may be local charities available to you too. Ask in your GP surgery for any that they can refer you to.

Glossary

Biotechnology

Biotechnology is the use of natural organisms and biological processes to change or manufacture products for human use. Biotechnology is widely used in modern society: for example, in agriculture, pharmaceuticals, the manufacturing industry, food production and forensics.

BMI (body mass index)

An abbreviation which stands for 'body mass index' and is used to determine whether an individual's weight is in proportion to their height. If a person's BMI is below 18.5 they are usually seen as being underweight. If a person has a BMI greater than or equal to 25, they are classed as overweight and a BMI of 30 and over is obese. As BMI is the same for both sexes and adults of all ages, it provides the most useful population-level measure of overweight and obesity. However, it should be considered a rough guide because it may not correspond to the same degree of 'fatness' in different individuals (e.g. a body builder could have a BMI of 30 but would not be obese because his weight would be primarily muscle rather than fat).

Cancer

Cancer is a disease in which some of the body's cells become abnormal and grow uncontrollably and can sometimes spread to other parts of the body. There are over 200 different types of cancer.

Cell

Cells are the basic building blocks of all living things. The human body is composed of trillions of cells, all with their own specialised function. A cell has three main parts: the cell membrane, the nucleus, and the cytoplasm.

Cervical cancer

Cancer that develops in a woman's cervix (the entrance to the womb from the vagina). In its early stages it often has no symptoms. Symptoms can include unusual vaginal bleeding which can occur after sex, in between periods or after menopause. The NHS offers a national screening programme; a 'smear test' for all women over 24 years old.

Genes

A gene is an instruction and each of our cells contains tens of thousands of these instructions. In humans, these instructions work together to determine everything from our eye colour to our risk of heart disease. The reason we all have slightly different characteristics is that before we are born our parents' genes get shuffled about at random. The same principles apply to other animals and plants.

Immune system

The immune system is made up of cells, tissue and organs that protect the body from viruses and infections. The HIV virus attacks the immune system and prevents the body from protecting itself.

NHS

The National Health Service provides free medical care to citizens of England, Scotland, Wales and Northern Ireland.

Oncologist

An oncologist is a doctor who treats cancer and provides medical care for a person diagnosed with cancer.

Oncology

Oncology is a branch of medicine that deals with the study, treatment, diagnosis and prevention of tumours.

Organ/tissue donation

The process of a person choosing to donate their organs/tissues for transplant. One donor can help several people because one person can donate a number of organs: kidneys, liver, heart, lungs, small bowel, pancreas, cornea (eye), bone, skin, heart valves, tendons and cartilage.

Palliative care

A specialist area of care which provides relief from pain but does not cure a disease or illness. It is often administered to patients suffering from terminal illnesses in order to improve their quality of life before they die.

Terminal illness

An illness for which there is no cure and which is likely to bring about the patient's death. Also known as a life-limiting illness.

Tumour

A tumour can be cancerous or benign. A cancerous tumour is malignant, meaning it can grow and spread to other parts of the body. A benign tumour means the tumour can grow but will not spread.

Index

A
additives 21
adults, common cancers 14
age 5, 7, 16, 17
alcohol 6, 10–11, 16
artificial sweeteners 19
asbestos 6
Australia 18

B
bacterial infections 7
benign tumours 1
bowel cancer 17
brain tumours 1–2, 8, 23
breast cancer 8, 26, 27
breast implants 20

C
campaigns, prevention 18
cancer, overview 1–3
carcinomas 1
causes 3, 19–21
cells 4, 12, 40–41
cervical cancer 31–32
checking for cancer 26–30
chemicals 6–7, 12, 19–21
chemotherapy 3, 34, 37–38
children 14–15
China 10–11
coffee 21
cosmetics 19–20

D
data gathering 15, 17
diagnosis rates 17
diet 6, 7, 8–9, 16, 19, 20–21
DNA damage 12
doctors, talking to 23, 24

E
environmental risk factors 7
exercise 6, 7, 16

F
family history 3, 5, 7

G
genes 4, 10–11

H
hepatitis B and C 7
high-dose treatments 34
HIV 7
Hodgkin lymphoma 22–23
hormonal therapy 34
hormones in cattle 20
human papilloma viruses (HPV) 7, 15, 32

I
immunity, low 7
immunotherapies 39–41

L
leukaemias 1
lifestyle 5–6, 16, 17
lung cancer 12–13, 17
lymphomas 1, 22–23

M
malignant tumours 2
meat 6, 17, 19, 20, 21
melanoma 18, 22, 29–30
mortality rates 17
mutations, cell 4

O
ovarian cancer 8, 23

P
pesticides 20
plastics 19
pre-cancerous conditions 7
prevention 16, 17, 18, 29, 31–32
prostate cancer 17

R
radiotherapy 3, 33–34
radon 7
risk factors 5–7

S
sarcomas 2
screening 16, 17, 31, 35–36
self-examination 26–30
side-effects of treatment 37–38
skin cancers 1, 18, 22, 29–30
smear tests 29
smoking 5, 7, 12–13, 16, 17
staging, cancer 2
stem cells 34
stress 19
sunlight (UV) 6, 7, 15, 16, 29
surgery 3, 33
survival rates 15
symptoms 2, 22–23, 24–25

T
T-cells 40–41
targeted therapies 34
testicular cancer 22, 26, 28
TNM (tumour, nodule, metastasis) system 2
toiletries 19–20
treatment 3, 33–34, 37–38, 39–41

U
ultra-processed foods 8–9

V
vaccines 32
vegan diet 19

viral infections 7

W
waiting times 35
water 21
weight 6, 7, 8–9, 16, 19
workplace risk factors 6–7

Y
young people 14–15, 22